PROMOTING PARTNERSHIP
FOR HEALTH

International Perspectives on Health and Social Care

Partnership Working in Action

PROMOTING PARTNERSHIP FOR HEALTH

International Perspectives on Health and Social Care

Partnership Working in Action

Edited by

Jon Glasby and Helen Dickinson

Health Services Management Centre,
University of Birmingham

Series editor: Hugh Barr

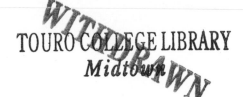

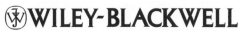

WILEY-BLACKWELL

A John Wiley & Sons, Ltd., Publication

CAIPE

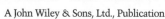

This edition first published 2009 by Blackwell Publishing Ltd
© 2009 by Blackwell Publishing Ltd

Blackwell Publishing was acquired by John Wiley & Sons in February 2007. Blackwell's publishing programme has been merged with Wiley's global Scientific, Technical, and Medical business to form Wiley-Blackwell.

Registered office
John Wiley & Sons Ltd, The Atrium, Southern Gate, Chichester, West Sussex, PO19 8SQ, United Kingdom

Editorial offices
9600 Garsington Road, Oxford, OX4 2DQ, United Kingdom
2121 State Avenue, Ames, Iowa 50014-8300, USA

For details of our global editorial offices, for customer services and for information about how to apply for permission to reuse the copyright material in this book please see our website at www.wiley.com/wiley-blackwell.

The right of the author to be identified as the author of this work has been asserted in accordance with the Copyright, Designs and Patents Act 1988.

Wiley also publishes its books in a variety of electronic formats. Some content that appears in print may not be available in electronic books.

Designations used by companies to distinguish their products are often claimed as trademarks. All brand names and product names used in this book are trade names, service marks, trademarks or registered trademarks of their respective owners. The publisher is not associated with any product or vendor mentioned in this book. This publication is designed to provide accurate and authoritative information in regard to the subject matter covered. It is sold on the understanding that the publisher is not engaged in rendering professional services. If professional advice or other expert assistance is required, the services of a competent professional should be sought.

Library of Congress Cataloging-in-Publication Data

International perspectives on health and social care : partnership working in action / edited by Jon Glasby and Helen Dickinson.
        p. ; cm. — (Promoting partnership for health)
    Includes bibliographical references and index.
    ISBN 978-1-4051-6743-7 (hardback : alk. paper)   1. Medical cooperation.   2. Interprofessional relations.   3. Social service.   I. Glasby, Jon.   II. Dickinson, Helen, 1979–   III. Series.
    [DNLM: 1. Partnership Practice.   2. Delivery of Health Care—organization & administration.   3. Interprofessional Relations.   4. Social Work—organization & administration.   W 92 I61 2008]

    R727.8.I58   2008
    610.69′6—dc22

                                                                                2008028182

A catalogue record for this title is available from the British Library

Set in 10/12.5 pt Palatino by Aptara® Inc., New Delhi, India
Printed in Singapore by Utopia Press Pte Ltd

1   2009

Contents

Contributors   vi
The Series   viii
Foreword   x
Acknowledgements   xii

Introduction   1
Helen Dickinson and Jon Glasby

1. Partnership working and organisational culture   10
   Edward Peck and Helen Dickinson

2. Interprofessional practice   27
   Celia Keeping and Gillian Barrett

3. Partnership working: key concepts and approaches   42
   Walter Leutz

4. Key elements in effective partnership working   56
   Henk Nies

5. Integrated service models: an exploration of North American models and lessons   68
   Dennis Kodner

6. Working across the health and social care boundary   81
   Amanda Edwards

7. Partnerships in the digital age   95
   Justin Keen and Tracy Denby

8. The economics of integrated care   107
   Marie-Eve Joël and Helen Dickinson

9. Self-management with others: the role of partnerships in supporting self-management for people with long-term conditions   121
   Gawaine Powell Davies, Sarah Dennis and Christine Walker

10. Self-directed support as a framework for partnership working   136
    John O'Brien and Simon Duffy

11. The outcomes of health and social care partnerships   152
    Helen Dickinson

Index   167

Contributors

About the editors

Jon Glasby is Professor of Health and Social Care and Co-Director of the Health Services Management Centre, University of Birmingham, UK.

Helen Dickinson is Lecturer in Health Care Policy and Management at the Health Services Management Centre, UK.

About the authors

Gillian Barrett is Senior Lecturer at the University of the West of England, UK.

Gawaine Powell Davies is Associate Professor and CEO of the University of New South Wales Centre for Primary Health Care and Equity, Australia.

Tracy Denby is Research Officer at the Leeds Institute of Health Sciences, University of Leeds, UK.

Sarah Dennis is Senior Research Fellow at the University of New South Wales Research Centre for Primary Health Care and Equity, Australia.

Simon Duffy is Chief Executive of in Control, a UK social enterprise, which has developed and rolled out the concept of an individual budget.

Amanda Edwards is Head of Knowledge Services at the UK's Social Care Institute for Excellence, a national body established to identify and disseminate good practice in UK social care. Amanda writes here in a personal capacity.

Chris Ham is Professor of Health Policy and Management at the Health Services Management Centre, University of Birmingham, UK.

Marie-Eve Joël is Professor of Health Economics at the Unit of Research in Health Economics, Dauphine University, Paris.

Justin Keen is Professor of Health Politics at the Leeds Institute of Health Sciences, University of Leeds, UK.

Celia Keeping is a part-time Social Work Practitioner and part-time Senior Lecturer at the University of the West of England, UK.

Dennis Kodner is Professor of Medicine and Gerontology at the New York College of Osteopathic Medicine of New York Institute of Technology (NYIT) and Director of the NYIT Center for Gerontology and Geriatrics, USA.

Walter Leutz is Associate Professor at Brandeis University, USA.

Henk Nies is Director of Vilans, Netherlands Centre of Expertise for Long-Term Care, Utrecht, the Netherlands.

John O'Brien is a member of the Center on Human Policy at Syracuse University.

Edward Peck is Professor of Public Service Development and Head of the College of Social Sciences, University of Birmingham, UK.

Christine Walker is Executive Officer at the Chronic Illness Alliance, Victoria, Australia.

The Series

Promoting partnership for health

Health is everybody's responsibility: individuals, families, communities, professions, businesses, charities and public services. It is more than prevention and cure of disease. It is life fulfilling for the well-being of all. Each party has its role, but effective health improvement calls for partnership, more precisely for many partnerships which bring them together in innovative and imaginative ways. The scope for this series is correspondingly wide.

Successive books explore partnership for health from policy, practice and educational perspectives. All drive change. Policy presses the pace of reform everywhere, but change is also driven by the demands of practice, triggered by economic and social trends, technological advance and rising public expectations. Education responds but also initiates as a change agent in its own right.

Progressive health care is client centred. The series will wholeheartedly endorse that principle, but the client is also relative, citizen, client and consumer:

- Relative sustaining, and sustained by, family
- Citizen working for, and benefiting from, community, country and comity of nations
- Client of countless professions
- Consumer of health-enhancing or health-harming services

A recurrent theme is the roles and responsibilities of professions, individually and collectively, to promote and sustain health. The focus will be on the health and social care professions, but taking into account the capability of every profession to improve or impair health. The responsibility of the professions in contemporary society will resonate throughout the series starting, from the premise that shared values of professionalism carry an inescapable obligation to further the health and well-being of all.

Each book will compare and contrast national perspectives, set within a global appreciation of opportunities and threats to health. Each will be driven, not simply by self-evident scope for one nation to learn from another, but also by the need to respond to challenges that pay no respect to national borders and can only be addressed by concerted action.

Partnership has become so fashionable that it is tempting to assume that all reasonable men and women will unite in common cause. Experience teaches otherwise: best-laid plans too often founder for lack of attention to differences which can bedevil relationships between professions and between organisations. This series is not starry eyed. It alerts readers to the pitfalls and to ways to avoid them.

This is the fourth book in the series. In the first, Meads *et al.* (2005) found collaboration critical to effective implementation of health care reforms around the world. In the second, Barr *et al.* (2005) made the case for interprofessional education as a means to promote collaborative practice corroborated by emerging evidence from systematic searches of the literature. In the third, Freeth *et al.* (2005) married evidence with experience to assist teachers to develop, deliver and evaluate interprofessional education programmes.

Hugh Barr
Series Editor
April 2008

References

Barr, H. *et al.* (2005) *Effective Interprofessional Education: Argument, Assumption and Evidence.* London, Blackwell Science.

Freeth, D. *et al.* (2005) *Effective Interprofessional Education: Development, Delivery and Evaluation.* London, Blackwell Science.

Meads, G. *et al.* (2005) *The Case for Interprofessional Collaboration.* London, Blackwell Science.

Foreword

Partnership working and inter-agency working are universal priorities and universal challenges. As the contributors to this volume show, the reasons are not hard to find. Changing needs driven by the ageing population and the increasing prevalence of chronic diseases call for a joined-up response. This has found expression in a series of demonstration projects and policy initiatives, starting with the PACE programme in the US and extending through Canada to Europe, Australasia and beyond. Evaluations of these projects have reported positive results, yet despite this they often remain on the margins of policy development. The evidence summarised here, drawing on experience from several countries and many disciplines, helps to explain why partnership working has struggled to enter the mainstream.

In his contribution (Chapter 3), Walter Leutz extends his seminal article on the five laws for integrating medical care and social care to illustrate the obstacles to progress. In part, these obstacles derive from the difficulty of achieving integration for all people all of the time, and in part they result from the time it takes to build integration. As he also notes, integration usually costs before it pays. Leutz helpfully distinguishes between different degrees of partnership working, ranging from linkage to coordination to full integration of services. As a pragmatist, his advice is to keep efforts at integration simple and not to attempt to integrate everything at once.

In Chapter 5, Dennis Kodner builds on Leutz's analysis and summarises the results of evaluations of three successful models that have achieved closer integration of care for frail older people in the US and Canada. Notwithstanding differences between the models, there are a number of factors that explain their success. Kodner emphasises in particular the contribution of umbrella organisational structures to guide integration, the role of case-managed, multidisciplinary team care in meeting client needs, the value of organised provider networks in delivering care and the use of financial incentives to promote prevention, rehabilitation and downward substitution of services. Looking at the future, he argues that integrated models of care have to go further to win acceptance and support from service users, above and beyond merely demonstrating positive results in terms of service utilisation or costs.

Some of the reasons why models that work fail to enter the mainstream are explored by other contributors. The importance of culture and differences in culture are highlighted by Edward Peck and Helen Dickinson (Chapter 1); the influence of professionals working together in teams and conflict between these professionals is explored by Celia Keeping and Gillian Barrett (Chapter 2); the importance and challenges of working across organisational and service boundaries are reviewed by Amanda Edwards (Chapter 6); the need for integration at different levels is discussed by Hank Nies (Chapter 4); and the potential of information technology to empower users to promote integration is analysed by Justin Keen and Tracy Denby (Chapter 7). Marie-Eve Joël and Helen Dickinson (Chapter 8) then review the economics of integrated care before the focus returns to the service user in contributions by Gawine Powell Davies, Sarah Dennis and Christine Walker on self-management (Chapter 9) and John O'Brien and Simon Duffy (Chapter 10) on self-directed support. Helen Dickinson (Chapter 11) concludes the book with a review of the issues involved in measuring outcomes of care.

In covering such a broad canvas in a readable and succinct manner, Glasby and Dickinson have succeeded in providing an accessible and comprehensive introduction to a topic that is bound to grow in significance. Students, teachers, practitioners and policy makers will all benefit from their careful and balanced exposition of the issues and the wealth of examples from different countries they have used to illustrate the argument. As they show, there are no short cuts to more effective partnership working, but there are many ways of making progress even in the face of adversity. The contributors to this book provide a solid foundation of empirical evidence and practical theory to help ensure that people most in need have access to high-quality integrated care.

Chris Ham
Professor of Health Policy and Management
Health Services Management Centre
University of Birmingham
UK

Acknowledgements

The editors are grateful to each of the authors, to Hugh Barr and to Katrina Chandler for all their help and support.

Chapter 5 of this book is an amended version of a journal article by the same author, which first appeared in *Health and Social Care in the Community* (2006), 14(5), 384–390. We are grateful to Blackwell and to *Health and Social Care in the Community* for their permission to reproduce this chapter.

Introduction

Helen Dickinson and Jon Glasby

When a new concept and a new way of working becomes prominent in most, if not all, developed countries at the same time, something fundamental happens. As the chapters in this edited collection attest, partnership working and inter-agency collaboration are an important and growing phenomenon in a number of different countries and continents, including North America, Western Europe, Australia and beyond. No matter how each system funds, organises and provides its welfare services, significant gaps and barriers exist, and greater coordination and collaboration remain a key aspiration. While the terminology used, the structures adopted and the chronology of policy change may vary, the underlying desire to create services that operate more effectively in conjunction with each other is equally strong. When one starts to look at the different contributions and perspectives in this book alone, some immediate questions arise: why this way of working and why now?

At face value, many individual countries justify their emphasis on partnership working in terms of a desire to create more seamless services and a better experience and outcome for people using such services. In the mantra of the UK New Labour government elected in 1997, for example, the aim is to create 'joined-up solutions to joined-up problems'. Open any policy document or consultation, and the potential pitfalls of the current (divided) system are contrasted with the perceived benefits of more coordinated or even integrated systems. A famous UK example comes from a 1998 government discussion paper on the future relationship between health and social care. Here, a typically forthright and explicit summary of the current situation was set out early on in the paper to pave the way for subsequent policy changes (Department of Health, 1998, p. 3):

> 'All too often when people have complex needs spanning both health and social care good quality services are sacrificed for sterile arguments about boundaries. When this happens people, often the most vulnerable in our society...and those who care for them find themselves in the no man's land between health and social services. This is not what people want or need. It places the needs of the organisation above the needs of the people they are there to serve. It is poor organisation, poor practice, poor use of taxpayers' money – it is unacceptable.'

The problem with this interpretation (that the emphasis on partnership working is a response to the desire to create better services) is that it does not explain the 'why now' dilemma. Historically, services have always experienced a degree of fragmentation, and it is not immediately clear why there should suddenly be such an emphasis on partnership working as a potential solution to *current* problems. Such an explanation also favours an interpretation of individual and organisational behaviour which assumes that it is possible to change practice through *the power of ideas*. Put simply, it is assumed that if any given government makes a powerful enough case for change, then change is likely to follow. In our experience, this is seldom the case, and the extent to which the 'power of ideas' can work depends on the extent to which there is a favourable climate for such ideas to be received. Thus, wider economic, political and cultural factors influence what it is possible to think and do at any given time. In this version of events, policy change depends not upon the charisma and vision of individual policy makers, but upon the current social context.

Against this background, we believe that the current emphasis on partnership working and inter-agency collaboration is based on at least three key factors (and there could well be more):

1. The impact of new public management (NPM) and the need to create greater coordination following the fragmentation of previous reforms
2. A recognition that partnership working is essential to respond to the challenges of individual organisations and the complexity of current social problems
3. The need to respond to a series of social changes (including a rise in the number of people with chronic or long-term conditions, technological advances and changing public expectations)

New public management

NPM reforms have been driven by a combination of economic, social, political and technological factors (see Larbi, 1999, for further exploration of these issues) and are broadly recognisable internationally – although the precise reform processes look slightly different within individual countries. The NPM view of bureaucracy is that it is inflexible and overly hierarchical. As such, the top-down decision-making processes associated with this model are increasingly distant from the expectations of citizens. NPM theorists drew on the commercial sector for lessons, arguing that because of the large-scale international competition that, private sector organisations had been exposed to from the 1980s onwards, those successful had become increasingly efficient whilst also offering consumers products which they wanted. While the commercial sector had undergone radical change, it was argued that, the public sector remained 'rigid and bureaucratic, expensive, and inefficient' (Pierre and Peters, 2000, p. 5).

The principles of NPM are, in general, characterised as an approach which emphasises output controls; disaggregates traditional bureaucratic organisations and decentralises management authority; introduces market and quasi-market mechanisms; and strives for customer-oriented services. This way of working puts much more emphasis on the importance of performance managing outcomes, determining what it is that service users want from their health and social care services and delivering this through flatter and less hierarchical structures. As Hood (1991) describes, these reforms are characterised by greater decentralisation of power to local levels, with managers increasingly taking responsibility for budgets and being allowed greater flexibilities in terms of their actions, but simultaneously bearing more responsibility for the outputs and outcomes of that particular unit. At the same time, NPM reforms have often led to services being delivered by a much larger range of providers (from the public, private and voluntary sectors), creating a subsequent need for greater coordination in order to reduce the negative implications of such fragmentation and congestion.

Complex social problems

Partnership working may be seen by some not to be driven purely by NPM reforms, but may in part arise due to the nature of the complex social problems which face societies within developed nations. These problems are recognised as 'wicked issues' (Rittel and Webber, 1973), that is, intractable social problems which no one individual agency, or indeed sector, would be able to address by acting independently. These wicked issues are not simply complex in terms of our ability to understand the range of processes at play, but also tend to be deep seated and temporally enduring issues which have not been effectively addressed (or even understood) by individual agencies in isolation. Organisations tend to work to their own specific agendas and are performance managed according to this, which might confound attempts to address these wicked issues. Such complex problems include hospital discharge planning, safeguarding children, long-term unemployment and particular types of criminal activity, all of which require a collaborative approach by multiple actors if they are to be effectively understood and resolved.

Social changes

It is well documented that there has been a marked shift in the types of problems which public services are facing, with chronic and complex health and well-being issues becoming ever more prevalent. Such conditions are much more resource intensive and require input over a longer time period than those traditionally faced by health and social care organisations. At the same time that these types of conditions have become more frequent, expectations about what public service organisations should be delivering and to what standard have also generally risen. Moreover, technological advancements mean that the range of available treatments and services has expanded and become ever more expensive. In a number of countries, health and social care services have become important vehicles through which successive governments have tried to demonstrate their effectiveness. These changes have been supplemented by a general trend in which the public have access to a number of different information sources and are becoming increasingly knowl-edgeable about a range of health and well-being issues. Consequently, service users and patients are becoming less comfortable in paternalistic relationships with ser-vice providers, and are more willing to challenge professionals and 'experts'. These changing expectations mean not only that agencies are required to collaborate with each other in order to share costs and deliver better-quality services, but also that they are increasingly required to enter into partnerships with the public and service users.

Overview of the book

Against this background, this edited collection adopts a thematic approach to health and social care partnerships. With chapters by leading international com-mentators, the book covers key partnership topics such as organisational culture, interprofessional practice, IT, economics and evaluating outcomes. While each in-dividual author comes from a specific national background, each chapter tries to place relevant national developments in an international context – using the na-tional mainly as a case study to explore a series of underlying themes and issues. After this initial introduction, Edward Peck and Helen Dickinson (Chapter 1) re-view the extensive literature on organisational and professional culture, drawing in particular on international lessons with regards to mergers and acquisitions (in both public and private sectors). While discussions about inter-agency working tend to focus on issues of process and structure, we believe that it is the per-sonal and the cultural issues that matter most – and these topics form the basis of the first two chapters in this book. Thus, Peck and Dickinson's opening contribu-tion is followed by a chapter from Celia Keeping and Gillian Barrett (Chapter 2), which explores the knowledge, attitudes and skills required for practitioners from different professional backgrounds to work together collaboratively. Key topics include issues such as power, trust, conflict and interprofessional education and training.

After this initial discussion of culture and of interprofessional practice, atten-tion shifts to more well-established debates about the principles and structures of partnership working. In Chapter 3, Walter Leutz (author of a famous article on the 'five laws of integration') explores some of the key concepts underpinning current approaches to partnership working and integration. Crucial to this analysis are three different ways of working together ('linkage', 'coordination' and 'full inte-gration', with each approach potentially more suitable for particular issues, service user groups and settings). So influential has Walter's initial and ongoing analysis been that many of the other chapters in this book also draw on and adapt these 'five laws'. Building on this, Chapter 4, by Henk Nies, draws on a range of sources (including an EU-funded study of services for older people in 11 EU countries) in order to identify and review the management of health and social care partner-ships and the organisational structures and infrastructure necessary to underpin effective joint working. Next, Dennis Kodner (Chapter 5) provides an overview of North American models of integrated service delivery, summarising some of the key approaches adopted, the outcomes achieved and the lessons learned. After this, Amanda Edwards summarises empirical research carried out in services for older people in Germany, Denmark, the US, Italy, the Netherlands and Australia (Chapter 6). Using the BIOSS (Brunel Institute of Organisational and Social Studies) tripod of work, this chapter summarises different approaches to inter-agency working and highlights a number of key lessons about the management of boundaries between health, social care and housing.

In Chapter 7, Justin Keen and Tracy Denby summarise and review current aspirations around the development of integrated IT systems, providing a hard-hitting and important critique of much recent policy and government thinking. While many accounts of IT systems focus on issues of confidentiality or on the problems associated with large public sector IT projects, this chapter explores the extent to which the development of new technology could transform the provision of health and social care (and even the notion of partnership working itself) or not. Next, Marie-Eve Joël and Helen Dickinson review the economic and financial implications of different types of integrated networks, identifying key lessons to date as well as areas requiring further research (Chapter 8). At this stage, the remainder of the book takes a slightly different turn, and the remaining three chapters focus in more detail on the issue of partnerships between services and service users. First, Gawaine Powell Davies and colleagues explore the concept of self-management, emphasising the way in which services need to engage with people with long-term conditions in new ways in order to respond to current and future social changes and demographic pressures within the health and social care system (Chapter 9). Next, John O'Brien and Simon Duffy review the development of individualised funding approaches and consumer-directed care, essentially exploring the extent to which this way of working may enable people to integrate their own 'care' by designing support that makes sense to them within the context of their own lives (Chapter 10). Finally, Helen Dickinson's chapter on evaluating health and social care partnerships seeks to explore the extent to which this way of working has produced new and better outcomes for service users in practice (Chapter 11). In particular, the chapter reviews a number of international examples of the types of partnership outcome indicators that have been developed and the findings of key studies to date.

Although the focus of many of the chapters in this book is on (often public sector) health and social care partnerships, we believe that the issues at stake relate to a range of different types of inter-agency and interpersonal relationships. As a result, we hope that the underlying themes in subsequent chapters will also be relevant to:

- inter-agency collaboration beyond health and social care;
- relationships between the public, private and voluntary sectors;
- relationships between formal services, family carers and people who use services.

While many individual contributors specialise in researching and writing about services for older people, we believe that the issues raised are relevant to other adult user groups (e.g. younger, disabled people, people with learning difficulties and people with mental health problems) as well as to some children and young people with cross-cutting needs.

As part of the Blackwell/CAIPE *Promoting Partnership for Health* series, this text is aimed at similar audiences to previous books in the current collection, including:

- masters-level and post-qualifying students in disciplines such as social work, nursing, allied health professions and medicine;
- academics and educators with an interest in joint working and interprofessional education;
- undergraduate modules on social policy programmes and professional training courses.

Because of its international focus, the book will also hopefully be relevant to readers in Western Europe, North America, Australia, New Zealand and beyond.

A note on terminology, language and design

With any edited collection, there is always a dilemma as to how best to balance individual expertise with the need for a consistent approach, feel and use of terms. This is even more complex in an international book, and becomes virtually impossible in a book on 'partnership working' – a phrase used by so many different people to refer to so many different types of relationships. As private individuals, we have often used the definition of collaboration adopted by Sullivan and Skelcher (2002), focusing on relationships in which partnerships are distinguished from other ways of organising services according to the extent to which they:

- involve negotiation between people from different agencies committed to working together over more than the short term;
- aim to secure the delivery of benefits or added value which could not have been provided by any single agency acting alone or through the employment of others (i.e. shared goals);
- involve the formal articulation of a purpose and a plan to bind partners together.

In particular, our own approach draws on two frameworks which we have often used to highlight the diversity of activity encompassed by notions of 'partnership' and to help readers to consider which way of working may be appropriate for which types of outcomes. In the first model (see Figure 1), partnership is seen as operating at a number of different levels of activity, with effective partnership working requiring a response at the individual, organisational and structural levels.

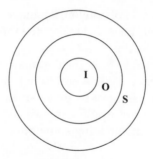

I: The individual level
O: The organisational level
S: The structural level

Figure 1 Understanding partnership working in health and social care (Glasby, 2003).

In the second model (see Figure 2), individuals and agencies working in partnership are given a series of options about the breadth and depth of the relationships that they need to establish in order to meet their desired outcomes.

However, these are very much personal preferences and models, and as editors, we have taken the (at times) uncomfortable step of enabling each individual author to adopt their own definition and employ their own terminology. Clearly, this runs the risk of creating an overall book in which the reader is pulled in too many different directions at once, but we feel that this approach is the best way of captur-

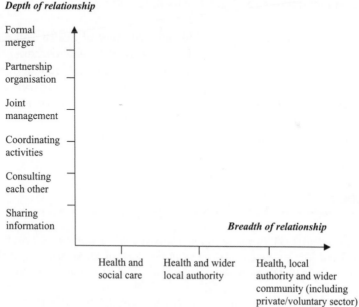

Figure 2 Depth versus breadth. (Adapted from Peck, 2002; see also Glasby, 2007.)

ing a flavour of the diversity of opinion, language and concepts that exist nationally and internationally. If at times this makes the topic feel messy and complex, then that is essentially because it is!

Similarly, we have tried to fight the temptation to standardise other key terms. In our view, the tendency of different authors to use different terms to refer to different concepts and user groups gives an insight into the broader approach adopted in their country of origin, and we have tried to emphasise the diversity of contributions by maintaining something of this diversity of language and approach.

Despite these caveats and editorial decisions, we have tried to give the remainder of the book as much coherence as possible by adopting a number of overarching approaches:

- We have asked each contributor to focus on a specific topic, but to include an appropriate mix of national and international commentary, analysis, references and further resources (for those interested in exploring specific issues in more detail).
- We have sought to encourage chapters that can act as stand-alone summaries of each topic, but which also cross-refer to each other as appropriate. Whilst this inevitably leads to a degree of repetition from time to time, we hope that this ultimately adds value due to the slightly different interpretations which individual authors often have of the same underlying issues and material.
- Wherever possible we have asked each author to adopt a similar structure, with an initial introduction to the issues at stake, a main body of text broken up by appropriate subheadings and a summary box of 8–10 key points, together with brief recommendations about further reading and relevant websites.

Overall, we hope what follows provides an overview of health and social care partnership working at a national and international level – perhaps ultimately demonstrating that for all different systems that do things differently, the underlying problems are often the same. While most systems are actively trying, they are still struggling to develop fully effective partnerships. Although we might continue to hope that one country has a magic answer that can be imported to make our own system function at maximum capacity, the contingency still seems a remote one.

References

Department of Health (1998) *Partnership in Action: New Opportunities for Joint Working between Health and Social Services – A Discussion Document*. London, Department of Health.

Glasby, J. (2003) *Hospital Discharge: Integrating Health and Social Care*. Abingdon, Radcliffe Medical Press.

Glasby, J. (2007) *Understanding Health and Social Care*. Bristol, Policy Press.

Hood, C. (1991) A public management for all seasons, *Public Administration*, 69, 3–19.

Larbi, G.A. (1999) *The New Public Management Approach and Crisis State*. UNRISD Discussion Paper No. 112, Switzerland.

Peck, E. (2002) Integrating health and social care, *Managing Community Care*, 10(3), 16–19.

Pierre, J. and Peters, B.G. (2000) *Governance, Politics and the State*. New York, St Martin's Press.

Rittel, H. and Webber, M. (1973) Dilemmas in a general theory of planning, *Policy Sciences*, 4, 155–169.

Sullivan, H. and Skelcher, C. (2002) *Working across Boundaries: Collaboration in Public Services*. Basingstoke, Palgrave.

1 Partnership working and organisational culture

Edward Peck and Helen Dickinson

In discussions of partnership working between health and social care agencies, one issue seems to recur more than any other: culture. Furthermore, it appears simultaneously to be both an aspiration for partnerships (e.g. to change culture) and an obstacle to partnerships (e.g. conflicts rooted in culture). This concurrent recognition of the importance of, and uncertainty about, culture is reflected in the huge volume of writings about culture in an organisational context where the term has many and varied definitions. As Scott and his colleagues (2003b) point out, '[U]nsurprisingly in view of this diverse array of phenomena, little agreement exists over a precise definition of organisational culture, how it should be observed or measured, or how different methodologies can be used to inform routine administration or organisational change' (p. 925). The aim of this chapter is to bring some clarity to discussions of culture in relation to partnership working.

Concern about culture in partnerships is not restricted to the public sector. There is compelling evidence from the private sector that culture is also a central issue in the success of alliances, mergers and acquisitions in the commercial field (see Field and Peck, 2003). Cartwright and Cooper (1996) have examined the cultural characteristics of companies and how these can affect the outcomes of mergers and acquisitions. They argue that the degree of 'cultural fit' can be critical in determining the outcome of a merger or an acquisition; they also suggest that most fail and that poor cultural fit between the new partners – leading to staff experiencing a loss of morale and a loss of commitment – is the main cause.

What do we mean by organisational culture?

Most accounts of culture assume what Meyerson and Martin (1987) call an *integration model*. This sees culture as something that organisations possess and which is therefore broadly recognisable and consistent across them. On this view, culture is an influence which promotes integration within organisations (thus two divergent cultures may need to be reconciled when organisations work in partnership) and may be manipulated in relatively predictable ways in order to enhance integration.

A few examples of this school of thought will establish its basic premises. One of the most frequently cited authors on organisations, Schein (e.g. 1985), suggests that organisational culture can be thought of as the shared basic assumptions that an organisation learns as it solves problems of adaptation and integration (or as Ouchi and Johnson, 1978, put it: 'the way we do things around here'). These assumptions are considered to be 'valid' and are taught to new members as the correct way to perceive, think, feel or act. There is broad agreement within the more thoughtful parts of this literature that organisational cultures are multi-layered, consisting of a central core that is overlaid with more superficial and easily influenced outer layers (e.g. Schein, 1985; Hofstede, 1991). The broad generalisations that such conceptions of culture generate can be very plausible (see Peck and Crawford, 2004, for more discussion of these in relation to health and social care).

A second approach identified by Meyerson and Martin (1987) conceptualises culture as more pluralistic, with disparate cultures being held by different interest groups within the same organisation. On this view, culture is an influence which may once again inhibit integration (and thus partnership), but where the various cultures may be open to manipulation, in particular in relation to the ways in which they interact. This is the *difference model* of culture.

Most health care organisations are composed of numerous and disparate professional cultures. Indeed, the mix of managerial and professional cultures in which multiple values coexist alongside power imbalances among the various staff groups has been seen as the key distinctive feature of the UK National Health Service (NHS) (Harrison *et al.*, 1992; Dawson, 1999). In such a context, there are risks in any attempt to develop a strong unitary culture which may overlook the richness within the pre-existing cultures and the complex meaning-making processes that they enable (Hawkins, 1997). Peck and Norman (1999) provide a summary of significant aspects of professional cultures as manifested in community mental health services in London in the late 1990s. This notion of difference – of defining who I am in distinction from who you are – is one of the key components of professional culture. It may not be one that it is wise to assume should always be challenged (e.g. boundaries between professionals should not necessarily be characterised as barriers to better services; see Peck *et al.*, 2001).

The third perspective discussed by Meyerson and Martin (1987) – the *ambiguity model* – considers culture to be more local and personal than the other two, constantly being negotiated and re-negotiated between individuals and groups within the organisation. These patterns of creation and re-creation of culture may be influenced by the organisation within which, and by the interest groups between which, they take place, but it is the one that perhaps offers the least prospect of predictable manipulation. Although this aspect may be the most opaque to observers, there was evidence from an evaluation of a mental health partnership between a health authority and a county council in the UK (Peck *et al.*, 2001) to support the importance of this level of culture in health and local government. There was considerable ambiguity around individual views of the trust and many staff felt that their relationship with other staff groups was largely dependent, as one employee put it, 'on the person'. On this account, culture is an enactment neither of organisational assumptions nor of professional subculture, but rather the ebb and flow of individual relationships.

In their study of partnership development in Somerset, Peck *et al.* (2001) identified the presence of all three of these levels of culture. Broadly, discussions with managers revealed an assumption of an integration model of culture, those with professional groups focused on professional difference and those with staff in localities suggested considerable negotiation and re-negotiation of culture, consistent with the ambiguity model. Clearly, therefore, deploying this framework has potential for aiding both interpretation of and intervention in culture. It is perhaps also worth noting that despite the language of partnership that runs through the research of Peck and his colleagues, this study focused on what is best described as a process of merger between health and social care.

It is also important to acknowledge the origins of the idea in anthropology, where the classical anthropological understanding of culture refers to institutionalised practices and accountabilities located within social structures (see Moore, 1997). Whether analysing whole societies or specific organisations, many anthropologists have argued that ideas and beliefs – the visible manifestations of culture – are to be explained by reference to the social structure in which they occur. Exploring this relationship between social structure and organisational culture in an English NHS Trust, Bate *et al.* (2000) describe the co-evolution of culture and structure, each shaping and in turn being shaped by the other. This link between culture and structure is clearly important for the discussion of culture in partnership organisations where the creation of new organisational forms inevitably changes the practices and accountabilities in ways that may be open to manipulation by managers.

The international evidence on culture in health and social care partnerships

The international health and social care partnership literature reflects the view that culture plays a vital role in creating effective partnerships. As suggested in the introduction to this chapter, this probably links to a wider private sector literature which proposes that culture plays an imperative part in the merger and acquisition process (e.g. Kilmann *et al.*, 1985; Bueno and Bowditch, 1989; Bijlsma-Frankema, 2001; see also Box 1.1 for key definitions). Private sector companies tend to put a large degree of effort into assessing and auditing the cultures of potential merger partners to check that it is compatible with their own (Dickinson *et al.*, 2006). What this implies is that culture is a 'component' that an organisation 'has' as an internal variable. Consequently, a number of typologies of cultures have been produced and are widely employed as they help 'make sense' of the organisation and typify the organisational 'style'. Such taxonomies usually comprise four elements (see, e.g., Handy, 1976; Pheysey, 1993; Schneider, 1994; Cartwright and Cooper, 1998) and are presumably so popular as they are simple to explain and make accessible to busy practitioners (Peck and Crawford, 2004).

Box 1.1   A note on terminology.

In this chapter we refer to mergers and acquisitions, particularly when drawing on literature from the private sector. This box gives an overview of what these two phenomena entail.

Mergers. Mergers intuitively seem to be a fairly simple concept. McClenahan and Howard (1999, p. 4) define a merger as 'the coming together into a single corporate body of two or more previously separate organisations'. However, Baskin *et al.* (2000) suggest a more complicated picture than this, stating that there are three different kinds of mergers:

  Partition. Managers assume that everything can continue as it has, with merged units operating side by side. This approach overlooks the tension that putting the units together may cause, and serious conflict results.

  Domination. One organisation and its culture take over another. This approach can often result in debilitating resentment in the 'defeated'.

  Synthesis. Through careful planning, design and execution, managers in the merging companies try to synthesise the best elements of each into a higher, superordinate harmony.

Furthermore, mergers may also be *horizontal* (i.e. companies with similar product types) or *vertical* (i.e. merger of a vendor and a customer). Therefore, although a merger is technically a coming together of two or more organisations, the depth and the extent to which these organisations merge may have very different connotations for the organisations in practice.

Acquisitions. An acquisition constitutes acquiring control of an organisation, usually called a target, by stock purchase or exchange. Like merger, this seems like a simple enough term in itself, but is made up of horizontal and vertical acquisitions, in the same way to mergers. There is also a further dimension regarding the mode of acquisition: hostile or uncontested. Hostile acquisitions, where the organisation is less than receptive to the proposal – often referred to as a *takeover*-tend to lead to less successful outcomes (Strower, 1998). However, some authors would argue that all mergers are acquisitions (McClenahan and Howard, 1999) due to the differing sizes of organisations and their relative resources. In the Introduction to this book, Glasby and Dickinson outlined the depth–breadth matrix, and this may be useful to use in thinking through where mergers and acquisitions sit in terms of other forms of partnership relationships.

The cultural typology literature stresses the danger of clashes of organisational culture on the grounds that it can lead to merger failure (Kilmann *et al.*, 1985; Chatterjee *et al.*, 1992; Atkinson, 2005). The literature suggests that organisations have such fundamentally different ways of framing issues, reacting to problems, enacting procedural rules and pursuing management styles that bringing such different cultures together can lead to a situation of 'us vs them' (Marks and Mirvis, 1992). Finding similar organisational cultures has become a common panacea for avoiding employee dissatisfaction – which could potentially undermine the success of a merger (Larsson, 1993). Ashkenas *et al.* (1998) provide a case study of a private company who walked away from a potential merger very late in proceedings – despite favourable financial prospects – on realising that differences in management cultures could make such a move very difficult. Many of these organisations use 'cultural audits' to identify any significant differences or similarities between core values, beliefs, attitudes and management styles of the organisations prior to change (Salama *et al.*, 2003).

Much of this literature stresses that enforced integration does not work. One partner is usually always dominant within partnership arrangements (even if only in size), and this could potentially instil a feeling of 'takeover' in one set of staff (McClenahan and Howard, 1999; see also Box 1.1). If the culture of the stronger party is imposed, it is suggested that tension, distrust and annoyance will result (Weber and Schweiger, 1992). A process of cultural audit is thought to guard against such a feeling of takeover; if aspects of good practice from both organisations are taken on by the new entity, then both can show that they have something positive to contribute to the process. Therefore, much of this literature assumes the integration model; by finding a partner with a similar culture, partnership working will be enhanced and any residual differences in culture can be manipulated.

However, although the issue of culture-fit is important, it is further suggested that too much 'fit' can reduce the synergetic effects expected from the merger process (Bijlsma-Frankema, 2001). Mergers are intended to produce effects which are bigger than the sum of the organisations involved in the process (much in the same way that health and social care partnerships are often promoted on the grounds that they produce synergy or 'collaborative advantage'; .Huxham and Vangen, 2005). In the private sector, mergers are thought to offer a good opportunity to challenge the assumptions and processes of individual organisations and find new and more effective ways of delivering services (Marks, 1997). If cultures are too similar, the product is effectively an extension of existing organisations, rather than the creation of some new and different entity.

Despite the importance that culture seems to have assumed within the public sector partnership literature, a surprisingly small proportion of the international literature discusses culture in anything more than a normative, coherent and unproblematic fashion. Although culture is frequently cited as an important factor within the process of partnership working, there is little consideration of what form precisely this factor takes (see, e.g., Hensing *et al.*, 1997; Hultberg *et al.*, 2002). Moreover, within these studies, culture tends to appear as somewhat of an afterthought: that is, post hoc, culture is suggested as the reason why the partnership was not as effective or did not conclude in the anticipated results (see, e.g., Timpka *et al.*, 1995; McCloughen and O'Brien, 2006). In other words after the event, the neglect of cultural factors is recognised as having played a potentially detrimental role in the effectiveness of the partnership.

In this way, the most common accounts from the international public sector partnership literature report the difference model of culture in practice, whilst operating under the assumption that an integration model would have created a more effective partnership. One such account is the report of an attempt to integrate health and social care management structures in the English boroughs of Barking and Dagenham. Wistow and Waddington (2006) report how this process ran into difficulties due to 'basic incompatibilities, largely derived from the mismatch in cultures' (p. 14). In the process, Wistow and Waddington summarise the characteristics of the NHS and social services partners (illustrated in Table 1.1). These are not uncommon characterisations of health and social care and relate in part to the differing professional 'models' of care which are frequently typified as underpinning health and social care.

In this case, the cultures are further described as being closely linked into the performance management systems and the national policy objectives which broadly frame these partners within much wider organisational contexts than the local area alone. It is suggested that these divergent underpinning expectations and values form an inherent barrier to creating partnerships between these organisations. Although local partners were not able to influence the separate NHS and local government accountability and priority-setting mechanisms, the research team suggest that more attention to changing cultures by identifying areas of differences and developing agreed strategies for managing them might have resulted in more effective partnership working. In this case, Wistow and Waddington suggest that too much attention was paid to the structure of the partnership, with insufficient attention paid to cultural factors. Thus, although the research from the locality suggests the difference model of culture, the researchers advocate an integration model in attempting to produce a more 'effective' partnership.

Writing from a Canadian perspective, Hall (2005) provides a historical overview of the growth of professional cultures – not only between health and social care organisations, but also intra-organisational differences in cultures – for example, between nurses and physicians. Some professional cultures are typified as possessing values which run counter to the spirit of collaboration due to the high value which they place on autonomy (Gage, 1998) and these constructions of culture largely cleave to the difference model (consonant with the findings of Peck and Norman, 1999). However, Hall argues that these differences not only pertain to the different models of health care underpinning these professions (as outlined earlier),

Table 1.1 Differences in characterisation of NHS and social services partners.

NHS	Social services
Treatment	Care
National targets	Local needs
Must dos	Local discretion
Universal services	Focus on vulnerable
Procedurally regimented and very top-down in style	Practical focus but has difficulty with strategy and planning

Adapted from Wistow and Waddington (2006, p. 14).

but also relate to deeply engrained factors such as class and gender. (Morrow *et al.*, 2005, also report similar findings in relation to multi-agency working in children's services.) In this way, the ambiguity model of culture is suggested and this is supported by Hojat *et al.* (2001) in a study of nurse–physician collaboration in the US and Mexico where the researchers demonstrate spatial and temporal variation in these professional cultures.

Similar conclusions are reached in Kharicha *et al.*'s (2005) study of general practitioner-attached social workers. Cultural differences are cited as existing between medical and social models, and these manifested themselves through a lack of understanding of and clarity over each other's roles, responsibilities, pressures and organisational procedures (often with regard to specific incidents). The researchers report a number of strategies which social workers used to overcome these difficulties, such as risk minimisation, conceding on policy and accepting pragmatic solutions, using nurses as mediators and resorting to hierarchical authority. Moreover, they report social workers expressing a real fear that by being absorbed into the practice teams, they would have difficulty working to social services priorities, agendas and entry criteria as they integrate into the culture. Therefore, although the social workers reported the difference model in terms of everyday practice, they were also acutely aware of the potential for the ambiguity model of culture to occur with its processes of negotiation and re-negotiation of cultures.

In addition to the Somerset example cited earlier, another study demonstrates the presence of all three models of culture. Cruser and Diamond (1996) studied a medical health programme at the Harris County Jail in the US. In this case mental health staff were placed into criminal justice settings, and the authors report clear professional *differences* between their cultures. The research team employed an organisational culture (OC) schema based on Diamond's theory of organisational cultures (Diamond, 1993). This schema contains four OC models, each of which defines the degree to which the mental health system takes responsibility for problems and solutions associated with offenders with mental impairments (illustrated in Figure 1.1). Each of the models represents a way of the partnership relating to the external environment as a manifestation of the way in which the mental health and criminal justice agencies are able to work together in partnership.

This approach suggests that the partners' abilities to interact with each other in understanding or being able to deal with the other's different value bases inform the culture of the partnership in its dealings with the outside world. According to this thesis, the institutional and autocratic models are isolated from the environment, the homogenised model is paralysed in its ability to interact with the environment but the resilient model is empowered to communicate with the environment. Although the OC model is used, Cruser and Diamond recognise that it is essentially a heuristic schema and that in practice culture is a product of individual self-systems and unconscious values may be more dynamic and diffuse than this 'ideal' type. In this way, Cruser and Diamond recognise the ambiguity model at the level of individual practice.

At the start of the project, the Harris County Jail was characterised as having a mixed OC model, and the partners related to each other differently in a number

Isolating - *Empowering*

INSTITUTIONAL MODEL	RESILIENT MODEL
Characteristics Mental health feels responsible for problems but unable to provide solutions. Culture is entrenched and defensive. Blame is externalised. Self-systems have diffuse boundaries. Multiple missions, pervasive anxiety and ritualistic behaviour exist.	**Characteristics** Mental health and criminal justice share responsibility for problems and solutions. Culture is collaborative and goal oriented. Beliefs and norms are constantly re-evaluated. Self-systems are mature and flexible. Mission is clear. Continuous quality improvement processes are integrated and active.
HOMOGENISED MODEL	AUTOCRATIC MODEL
Characteristics Neither system takes responsibility for problems or solutions. Culture is inattentive to surroundings. Self-systems suppress leadership. Roles and rules are unclear. Individuals suppress thoughts and feelings, avoid communication, and see their group as good, others as bad.	**Characteristics** Mental health feels responsible for solution and externalises blame for the problem. Culture is leader controlled with suppressed group identity. Self-systems are aggressor like. Staff seek freedom from leader control. Tasks take precedence over mission. Independent thinking is not tolerated.

Paralysing - *Isolating*

Figure 1.1 The organisational culture schema. (Adapted from Cruser and Diamond, 1996, p. 141.)

of different parts of the system. However, the management brought in a series of changes to the environment, leadership, human resources management, training and roles of staff members in an attempt to alter the OC model to a fully resilient model – that is the management assumed an integration model in an attempt to modify the culture of the partnership.

What interventions shape culture?

There are a number of messages from the international literature which are important in thinking about interventions in culture. Most strikingly, it is clear that culture becomes particularly important when a merger of two (or indeed more) cultures is proposed; indeed, two key questions arise.

Firstly, is the management of culture possible? It appears that the difference and ambiguity views of culture offer less hope to the would-be manipulators of culture than the integration model. Parker (2000) offers two conclusions from his review of the culture literature (and his case studies based in health care settings): the first is that 'cultural management in the sense of creating an enduring set of shared beliefs is impossible' (p. 228); on the other hand, he suggests that 'it seems perverse to argue that the "climate", "atmosphere", "personality", or culture of an organisation cannot be consciously altered' (p. 229). This is broadly the view adopted in the rest of this chapter, although it also acknowledges – along with Bate *et al.* (2000) – the poor track record of corporate cultural change programmes that do not simultaneously look at the prospects for changes in practices and accountabilities where social structures are also amended.

Secondly, is structural change, therefore, enough to change culture? It would appear that structural change – the predominant tool for cultural change in Somerset, for example – may not be enough; the creation of a partnership trust (and associated innovations such as the co-location of health and social care staff) was not in itself a sufficient condition to create the desired cultural changes during the first 3 years (albeit that might be an optimistic timeframe within which to expect such changes). Indeed, in the short-term at least, structural change may have served to strengthen attachment to existing professional cultures (see Peck *et al.*, 2002). With these caveats in mind, this section now examines a range of tools for and approaches to interventions in culture in organisations.

In a systematic review of quantitative measures of organisational culture that have either been validated and used in health care settings or appear to have potential for use in such settings, Scott *et al.* (2003b) identify a total of 13 instruments (illustrated in Box 1.2). Scott and his co-authors (2003a) argue for the pragmatic selection of an instrument based on the purpose and context of any assessment. They identify four things to think about in utilising these tools:

- *Levels* (i.e. are you looking at the central core or more superficial manifestations?)
- *Triangulation* (i.e. are you drawing messages following comparisons of data from various sources?)
- *Sampling* (i.e. are you asking a representative number of staff?)
- *Analysis* (e.g. are you going to explore the results by professional group or by geographical locality?)

In an account of an intervention in the creation of a care trust (i.e. an integrated English health and social care organisation), Peck and Crawford (2004; see also Peck and 6, 2006) report on the use of a specifically designed cultural audit tool. The aim of the intervention was to establish perceptions of existing NHS and social services organisational cultures and aspirations for the organisational culture within the care trust. It is perhaps telling the extent to which staff identified innovations in the social structure (e.g. supervision arrangements and IT systems) as central to the delivery of their cultural aspirations for the care trust; it appears that staff already recognised the importance of the interplay between structure and culture as discussed by Bate and colleagues (2000). At the same time, there were some suggestions – such as creating a 5-year vision for the merged organisation – that were not dependent on structure at all. Furthermore, the managers took to heart one of the key messages in the 'culture cookbooks' on mergers:

Box 1.2   Quantitative organisational culture measures.

Typological approaches:

- Competing values questionnaire
- Harrison's organisational ideology questionnaire
- Quality improvement implementation survey

Dimensional approaches:

- Organisational culture inventory
- Hospital culture questionnaire
- Nursing unit culture assessment tool
- Practice culture questionnaire
- MacKenzie's culture questionnaire
- Survey of organisational culture
- Corporate culture questionnaire
- Core employee opinion questionnaire
- Hofstede's organisational culture questionnaire
- Organisational culture survey

After Scott *et al.* (2003b).

---

that staff from the two agencies merging should be given as many opportunities as possible to meet in so-called transitional groups to explore preconceptions and perspectives (see Peck and Smith, 2006, for a discussion of this and other messages).

Of course, this cultural analysis was itself an intervention in culture. As one consequence, staff reflected on the changes in culture that they wanted to see addressed through alterations in social structure; many of these focus on the assumptions that divide health care from social care and profession from profession. The very process of such reflection can be assumed to have generated some commitment to change; certainly, it highlighted for managers the issues where staff wanted them to take action and simultaneously created some legitimacy for such action. Overall, Dickinson *et al.* (2007) conclude that leaders in this case study adopted an integrationist view of culture. In doing so, consistency remained a key message to staff throughout this organisational transition and the change did not appear to cause the distraction to core business which the literature suggests it would. However, this continuity may have come at a cost, at least initially. In the process of formalising the previous partnership into a care trust, these leaders may not have produced all the beneficial effects of synergy which are usually (albeit eventually) associated with mergers in the private sector. Certainly, local actors could see opportunities that had been missed. This study serves to confirm that the integrationist conception of culture is limited and that the differentiation of professional groupings and the ambiguity of individual experience will always make contested the meanings that are attributed to organisational change.

Nonetheless, local leaders acknowledged the perceived threat to social care values arising from the location of social care staff in health settings which was expressed as clearly in this locality as it was in the research of Peck and Norman (1999). To address this concern, managers identified one of the central cultural issues for social care staff as relating to the response to diversity; the core assumption of social care is that the negative life experiences of clients should be challenged and the manifestation is that social care staff must receive training in anti-discriminatory practice. As a consequence, all new recruits to the care trust – regardless of professional background – receive such training as part of their induction. Of course, such training may not overcome counter-cultural values and assumptions held by either professions or individuals, but this initiative has both an instrumental and a symbolic purpose that is viewed as crucial to the care trust culture manifesting social care values and assumptions.

As suggested in the Introduction to this chapter, a number of commentators from the commercial sector (e.g. Cartwright and Cooper, 1996) have suggested that the majority of mergers and acquisitions fail in practice. Such commentators typically define the degree of success or failure predominantly within financial terms, yet suggest that the reason for this failure is a preoccupation with structures at the expense of the 'human factor' (culture). However, this may in fact be a false dichotomy. Peck and 6 (2006) suggest that the divergent institutional practices and accountabilities around budgeting arrangements and performance management of financial targets that impact upon health and social care agencies (as also demonstrated by Wistow and Waddington, 2006; see earlier) are a major influence on the cultures of the partners so that cultural and financial issues are closely intertwined. This is further demonstrated through Johri et al.'s (2003) study of international experiments with integrated care. The team looked at integrated care programmes and demonstrations from the UK, the US, Italy and Canada and draw common features of effective integrated care from these case studies. One of the critical features of these programmes is the use of financial levers (see also Chapter 5). Typically, this is exemplified by the integrated care programme taking responsibility for a set of risks associated with working together, but with the financial rewards should they save money through appropriate downward substitution (e.g. in the case of care of older people, reducing institutional expenditure through supporting individuals within their own homes).

Partnership working has a tendency to be predicated on a notion that it will improve outcomes for those that use services (see Chapter 11 for further discussion) and as such issues of finance tend to be much less discussed – publicly and rhetorically at least. However, this chapter argues that partnership culture is in part shaped by and intertwined with not only the structures but also the institutional arrangements of partners. Thus, any attempts to intervene or shape culture must take account of these factors within fairly wide contexts.

Conclusion

It is apparent that health and social care organisations – and their staff – approach new partnership arrangements (be they genuine partnerships, mergers or, indeed, acquisitions) with well-established perceptions – both positive and negative – of each other. These perceptions, and in particular the points of tension, are often expressed in terms of culture. Further, it is clear that culture plays a major role in the success or failure of partnerships. The process of creating and sustaining new partnership forms between health and local government thus needs to pay careful attention to culture.

The management literature contains many examples of claimed 'makeovers' of organisational culture (e.g. Shirley, 2000; Bernick, 2001), and these may prove illuminating to those seeking to address organisational dysfunction apparently rooted in poor fits between cultures. Yet, the claims of the champions of culture as a tool for integration are often overstated and the potential for interventions to have a transformational effect on organisational culture(s) is limited. It is for these reasons that Davies *et al.* (2000) urge a cautious reassessment of the possibilities for cultural transformation in the UK NHS which would involve sensitivity to subcultural differences, honouring current achievements and consideration of the needs, fears and motivations of diverse staff groups. Nonetheless, Ogbonna and Harris (2000), following Martin (1985), argue that organisational culture cannot be managed *but* may be manipulated under specific contingencies (including the formation of an organisation, periods of crisis and during leadership turnover). This seems a plausible conclusion, consistent with the position of most thoughtful commentators (e.g. Parker, 2000), and one that highlights the opportunities that face managers and practitioners during the creation of partnership arrangements and organisations.

Of course, any health and social care partnership is working with several professional cultures – with difference – as well as with (at least) two organisational cultures. Regardless of the organisational form chosen, any strategy to manipulate organisational culture in health and local government will have to work with, and through, these professionals and their cultures. In these circumstances, managers should not be lured by the culture cookbooks into assuming that all tension deriving from cultural difference within organisations is either unhealthy and/or avoidable. At the same time, Bate *et al.* (2000), and the case study in the preceding section, draw attention to the importance of innovations in social structure in potentially mediating the impact of these cultures.

Finally, is there a clear link between organisational culture and organisational performance? From their exhaustive study in health care, Scott *et al.* (2003b) decide that empirical studies do not provide clear answers, whilst noting that the available research is small in quantity, mixed in quality and variable in methodology (thus making comparisons between studies difficult). This is of course very different to the confident assertions of the authors of the culture cookbooks. However, it seems counter to our intuition and our experience to deny any such link, challenging as this may be to prove to the satisfaction of researchers. Ultimately, consideration of both the literature and previous experience suggests that through reflecting on and intervening in organisational culture(s) with sense and sensitivity, partially through re-designing social structures when opportunities arise, managers and practitioners can achieve some change in that culture, whilst being aware that such interventions may well have unanticipated aspects.

Summary

- In discussions of partnership working between health and social care, one issue seems to recur more than any other: culture.
- There is compelling evidence that culture is also a central issue in the success of alliances, mergers and acquisitions in the commercial field. In this context it is often suggested that mergers and acquisitions fail due to the precedence of structural over human (cultural) factors.
- Culture is a complex concept with many different underpinning models suggested by various commentators, but typically tends to be treated in a rather normative or coherent fashion in practice.
- Meyerson and Martin's (1987) distinction between three models of culture (integration, difference and ambiguity) is useful in thinking about concepts of culture within a partnership context.
- The commercial sector (and a number of management 'cookbooks') tend to point to the importance of 'culture-fit' and suggest tools such as cultural audits to make mergers and acquisitions 'work'. However, there is a danger that too much fit might reduce the synergetic effects associated with mergers.
- In the public sector, different professional values, models of care and performance management and regulatory systems are all illustrated as factors which inform differing health and social care cultures and form barriers to partnership working. However, it cannot be assumed that breaking these down is necessarily the most effective tactic to overcome these differences.
- Structural change alone seems to be an insufficient condition to create cultural change. Indeed, in the short-term at least, structural change may serve to strengthen attachment to professional cultures.
- There is little empirical evidence from health and social care linking culture and organisational performance, although implicitly it seems likely that there is some form of association.
- Organisational culture change may be achieved partially through redesign of social structures, but such interventions may also have impacts which are not predicted at the outset.

Further reading and useful websites

Useful texts include:

Bate P. (1995) *Strategies for Cultural Change*. Oxford, Butterworth-Heinemann.

Meyerson, D. and Martin, J. (1987) Cultural change: an integration of three different views, *Journal of Management Studies*, 24, 623–643.

Parker, M. (2000) *Organisational Culture and Identity*. London, Sage.

Schein, E. (1985) *Organizational Culture and Leadership*. San Francisco, Bass.

Relevant websites include:

The Integrated Care Network has publications supporting partnership and integrated working within the UK, including a discussion paper on culture and partnership working: http://www.integratedcarenetwork.gov.uk

Aston Organisation Development is a spin out company from Aston Business School that hosts a wealth of resources and information focused on the evidence around effective team-based working: (http://www.astonod.com/index.php)

Inter-logics is a multidisciplinary consulting practice specialising in work with complex organisations and multi-agency partnerships: (http://www.inter-logics.net/default.aspx)

References

Ashkenas, R.N., DeMonaco, L.J. and Francis, S.C. (1998) Making the deal real: how GE Capital integrates acquisitions, *Harvard Business Review*, 7, 165–178.

Atkinson, P. (2005) Managing resistance to change, *Management Services*, 14–19.

Baskin, K., Goldstein, J. and Lindberg, C. (2000) Merging, de-merging, and emerging at Deaconess Billings Clinic, *Physician Executive*, 26, 20–26.

Bate, P., Khan, R. and Pye, A. (2000) Towards a culturally sensitive approach to organizational structuring: where organization design meets organization development, *Organization Science*, 11, 197–211.

Bernick, C.L. (2001) When your culture needs a makeover, *Harvard Business Review*, 79, 53–61.

Bijlsma-Frankema, K. (2001) On managing cultural integration and cultural change processes in mergers and acquisitions, *Journal of European Industrial Training*, 25, 192–207.

Bueno, A.F. and Bowditch, L. (1989) *The Human Side of Mergers*. San Francisco, Jossey-Bass.

Cartwright, S. and Cooper, C.L. (1996) *Managing Mergers, Acquisitions and Strategic Alliances: Integrating People and Culture*. Woburn, MA, Butterworth-Heinemann.

Cartwright, S. and Cooper, C.L. (1998) Company cultures in M&A, *The Antidote*, 3, 31–33.

Chatterjee, S. *et al.* (1992) Cultural differences and shareholder value in related mergers: linking equity and human capital, *Strategic Management Journal*, 7, 119–140.

Cruser, D.A. and Diamond, P.M. (1996) An exploration of social policy and organizational culture in jail-based mental health services, *Administration and Policy in Mental Health*, 24, 129–148.

Davies, H.T., Nutley, S. and Mannion, R. (2000) Organisational culture and quality of health care, *Quality in Health Care*, 9, 111–119.

Dawson, S. (1999) Managing, organising and performing in health care: what do we know and how can we learn? in A. Mark and S. Dopson (eds) *Organisational Behaviour in Health Care*. London, Macmillan.

Diamond, P.M. (1993) *The Unconscious Life of Organizations: Interpreting Organizational Identity*. Westport, CT, Quorum Books.

Dickinson, H., Peck, E. and Davidson, D. (2007) Opportunity seized or missed? A case study of leadership and organizational change in the creation of a care trust, *Journal of Interprofessional Care*, 21, 503–513.

Dickinson, H., Peck, E. and Smith, J. (2006) *Leadership in Organisational Transition – What Can We Learn from Research Evidence? Summary Report*. Birmingham, Health Services Management Centre.

Field, J. and Peck, E. (2003) Mergers and acquisitions in the private sector: what are the lessons for health and social services? *Social Policy and Administration*, 37, 742–755.

Gage, M. (1998) From independence to interdependence, *Journal of Nursing Administration*, 28, 17–26.

Hall, P. (2005) Interprofessional teamwork: professional cultures as barriers, *Journal of Interprofessional Care*, May, 188–196.

Handy, C. (1976) *Understanding Organizations*. London, Penguin.

Harrison, C. *et al.* (1992) *Just Managing: Power and Culture in the National Health Service*. London, Macmillan.

Hawkins, P. (1997) Organizational culture: sailing between evangelism and complexity, *Human Relations*, 50, 417–441.

Hensing, G., Timpka, T. and Alexandersson, K. (1997) Dilemmas in the daily work of social insurance officers, *Scandinavian Journal of Social Welfare*, 6, 301–309.

Hofstede, G. (1991) *Cultures and Organisations: Software of the Mind*. London, McGraw-Hill.

Hojat, M. *et al.* (2001) Attitudes toward physician–nurse collaboration: a cross-cultural study of male and female physicians and nurses in the United States and Mexico, *Nursing Research*, 50, 123–128.

Hultberg, E.-L., Lonnroth, K. and Allebeck, P. (2002) Evaluation of the effect of co-financing on collaboration between health care, social services and social insurance in Sweden, *International Journal of Integrated Care*, 2. Available online via www.ijic.org

Huxham, C. and Vangen, S. (2005) *Managing to Collaborate: The Theory and Practice of Collaborative Advantage*. Abingdon, Routledge.

Johri, M., Béland, F. and Bergman, H. (2003) International experiments in integrated care for the elderly: a synthesis of the evidence, *International Journal of Geriatric Psychiatry*, 18, 222–235.

Kharicha, K. *et al.* (2005) Tearing down the Berlin wall: social workers' perspectives on joint working with general practice, *Family Practice*, 22, 399–405.

Kilmann, R.H., Saxton, M.J. and Serpa, R. (1985) *Gaining Control of the Corporate Culture*. San Francisco, Jossey-Bass.

Larsson, R. (1993) Barriers to acculturation in mergers and acquisitions: strategic human resource implications, *Journal of European Business Education*, 2(2), 1–18.

Marks, M.L. (1997) Consulting in mergers and acquisitions: interventions spawned by recent trends, *Journal of Organizational Change*, 10, 267–279.

Marks, M.L. and Mirvis, P.H. (1992) Rebuilding after the merger: dealing with 'survivor sickness', *Organizational Dynamics*, 21(2), 18–32.

Martin, J. (1985) Can organizational culture be managed? in P. Frost, *et al.* (eds) *Organizational Culture*. London, Sage.

McClenahan, J. and Howard, L. (1999) *Healthy Ever After? Supporting Staff through Merger and Beyond*. Abingdon, Health Education Authority.

McCloughen, A. and O'Brien, L. (2006) Interagency collaborative research projects: illustrating potential problems, and finding solutions in the nursing literature, *International Journal of Mental Health Nursing*, 15, 171–180.

Meyerson, D. and Martin, J. (1987) Cultural change: an integration of three different views, *Journal of Management Studies*, 24, 623–643.

Moore, J.D. (1997) *Visions of Culture: An Introduction to Anthropological Theories and Theorists*. London, AltaMira.

Morrow, G., Malin, R. and Jennings, T. (2005) Interprofessional teamworking for child and family referral in a Sure Start local programme, *Journal of Interprofessional Care*, 19, 93–101.

Ogbonna, E. and Harris, L.C. (2000) Leadership style, organizational culture and performance: empirical evidence from UK companies, *The International Journal of Human Resource Management*, 11, 766–788.

Ouchi, W. and Johnson, A. (1978) Types of organisational control and their relationship to organisational well-being, *Administrative Science Quarterly*, 23, 292–317.

Parker, M. (2000) *Organisational Culture and Identity*. London, Sage.

Peck, E. and Crawford, A. (2004) *'Culture' in Partnerships – What Do We Mean by It and What Can We Do About It?* Leeds, Integrated Care Network.

Peck, E., Gulliver, P. and Towell, D. (2002) *Modernising Partnerships: An Evaluation of Somerset's Innovations in the Commissioning and Organisation of Mental Health Services*. London, Institute of Applied Health and Social Policy, King's College.

Peck, E. and Norman, I.J. (1999) Working together in adult community mental health services: exploring inter-professional role relations, *Journal of Mental Health*, 8, 231–242.

Peck, E. and 6, P. (2006) *Beyond Delivery: Policy Implementation as Sense-Making and Settlement*. Basingstoke, Palgrave Macmillan.

Peck, E. and Smith, J. (2006) A bit of a blur? How to handle change, *Health Service Journal*, 116, 22–23.

Peck, E., Towell, D. and Gulliver, P. (2001) The meanings of 'culture' in health and social care: a case study of the combined trust in Somerset, *Journal of Interprofessional Care*, 15, 319–327.

Pheysey, D. (1993) *Organizational Cultures: Types and Transformations*. London, Routledge.

Salama, A., Holland, W. and Vinten, G. (2003) Challenges and opportunities in mergers and acquisitions: three international case studies – Deutsche Bank-Bankers Trust; British Petroleum-Amoco; Ford-Volvo, *Journal of European Industrial Training*, 27, 313–321.

Schein, E. (1985) *Organizational Culture and Leadership*. San Francisco, Bass.

Schneider, W. (1994) *The Reengineering Alternative: A Plan for Making Your Current Culture Work*. Oxford, Radcliffe Press.

Scott, T. *et al.* (2003a) *Healthcare Performance and Organisational Culture*. Oxford, Radcliffe Medical Press.

Scott, T. *et al.* (2003b) The quantitative measurement of organisational culture in health care: a review of the available instruments, *Health Services Research*, 38, 923–945.

Shirley, J. (2000) Clinical governance in an independent hospital, *Clinician in Management*, 9, 229–233.

Strower, M.L. (1998) M&A: not for the average company? *The Antidote*, 8–9.

Timpka, T., Hensing, G. and Alexandersson, K. (1995) Dilemmas in sickness certification among Swedish physicians, *European Journal of Public Health*, 5, 215–219.

Weber, Y. and Schweiger, D.M. (1992) Top management culture conflict in mergers and acquisitions: a lesson from anthropology, *The International Journal of Conflict Management*, 3, 285–302.

Wistow, G. and Waddington, E. (2006) Learning from doing: implications of the Barking and Dagenham experiences for integrating health and social care, *Journal of Integrated Care*, 14, 8–18.

2 Interprofessional practice

Celia Keeping and Gillian Barrett

Following on from earlier discussions of organisational culture, this chapter uses a fictional UK case study (see Box 2.1) to explore some of the factors that impact upon collaborative relationships between those at the front-line of interprofessional practice. While it is of course necessary to address practical constraints to partnership working such as complicated joint funding arrangements or incompatible IT systems (for the latter, see Chapter 7), steps to address such issues are not in themselves sufficient to ensure coordinated practice. Hudson and Henwood (2002) in their review of partnership working acknowledge the importance of

---

Box 2.1   Gerry's story.

Gerry pursued a successful career as an architect, living independently and enjoying an active social life. Despite a stable family background, his mental health was variable and he suffered from elements of an obsessive-compulsive disorder. At one point in his young adult life, he suffered a 'breakdown' requiring hospital treatment and he decided to return to live with his parents. Things did not go well with Gerry and his compulsive behaviour continued and led him to one day drink so much water that he collapsed and came near to death. He survived, yet suffered irreversible brain damage. His powers of comprehension were significantly reduced and his speech deteriorated drastically. He was unable to care for himself on a personal, practical or financial level, and he became very childlike in his behaviour and interests.

Gerry was initially cared for in a hospital 200 miles away from his parents. He was very unhappy there and his continual attempts to run away led to him being placed on a compulsory hospital order. Gerry wanted more than anything to live with his parents but this was impossible as they were by now elderly and in poor health and, despite their deep concern for their son, were unable to care for him in their home.

In considering the need for Gerry to live near his parents and given the absence of suitable residential care, it was decided to set up a package of care which would enable Gerry to live in his own home close to his parents.

addressing organisational structures and boundaries, but believe that these steps alone do not guarantee good collaborative working. Some of the perhaps more intractable and certainly less visible factors influencing interprofessional working relate to the relationships of those involved (see also Chapter 1 for further discussion) – particularly in situations when pressures on front-line workers and staff stress may prevent practitioners from collaborating as much as they would like. Psychological dynamics have a significant part to play in the ability of groups of people to work together effectively and are central to effective inter-agency working.

The interprofessional team

In Gerry's case the social worker from a Community Mental Health Team in his hometown was responsible for setting up his care package and she thus took on the role of care coordinator. Her starting point was a holistic assessment of Gerry's needs, the complexity of which meant that his requirements were beyond the scope of any one professional. An interprofessional response was therefore required involving staff from a number of public, private and voluntary agencies (see Box 2.2). As indicated within the case study, interprofessional working can involve a wide range of different professionals each with their own unique perspective and established working practices. This complex mix of relationships does not always run smoothly for a variety of reasons, some of which are discussed below.

Box 2.2   Gerry's story continued.

Setting up a package of care for Gerry entailed firstly obtaining public housing through the Housing and Social Services Department of the local authority. The resulting flat needed furnishing which involved further negotiations with the Housing Department and local voluntary agencies. Gerry required 24-hour care and an independent domiciliary care agency was commissioned to provide this. The funding of this arrangement fell largely on the local authority via the social services budget, but also the local Primary Care Trust (i.e. the local provider and commissioner of primary and community health services) and a central government-organised fund called 'Supporting People'.

Gerry also required ongoing medical support which was provided by his general practitioner and the consultant psychiatrist as well as specific help with his compulsive disorder from the clinical psychologist. He also needed activities which were provided by various voluntary sector organisations. Meanwhile, Gerry had his own informal network of support which consisted largely of his parents, brother and members of his local church.

Conflict

Despite the rhetoric and the sometimes glib pronouncements about getting beyond a 'silo mentality' and engaging in 'joined up thinking and action', interprofessional working has encountered many difficulties (Glasby and Lester, 2004). In the UK, the tendency towards idealism by the Blair government resulted in the vision of a workforce where the process of social change was unimpeded by the 'dark side' of human nature. Hoggett (2004) argues, however, that conflict is inherent within all social relationships and indeed is even necessary if social bonds are to be any more than superficial 'fronts' masking underlying tensions and ultimate disintegration. The German sociologist, George Simmel (1955), believed that relationships within society are complicated by dynamics which are hard to identify yet have far-reaching influence on the ability of people to cooperate and work collaboratively. Social solidarity in all areas of public life is thus a much more 'messy' and potentially disturbing business than the straightforward consensual process of collaborative working portrayed by policymakers. As Cooper and Lousada (2005) point out: 'there is something very persecuting about being *told* [their italics] to have relationships, as if making friends and partners was easy' (p. 116). In order to understand the nature of possible conflict between those involved in interprofessional working, it is useful to refer to the case study (see Box 2.3).

In his study of working relationships between two different psychiatric teams, Mattieu Daum coined the term 'relationship-in-the-mind' (Daum, 2002). This term describes the psychological experience of a relationship and acknowledges that it will consist of both conscious and unconscious elements. Daum argues that relationships between individuals and groups are largely 'imagined' phenomena as they are so greatly influenced by psychological factors. This chimes with the work of Benedict Anderson (1983) and has been taken up by many social theorists who believe that all communities, be they country, city, ethnic or occupational group, are most importantly imagined communities. By this we mean that whatever the realities of a group, community or society, we impose our own picture, driven by our own needs, of what that community is like, and thus how we relate to it.

The processes involved in misunderstanding and conflict such as that seen between the social worker and the psychologist can be explained by psychoanalysis, a theory which maintains that the unconscious is a powerful agent in human relationships. It argues that in order to deal with difficult and hard to bear feelings, individuals commonly resort to a primitive defensive process whereby those feelings causing anxiety are unconsciously split off and located or *projected* onto another individual, or group of individuals. The person is thus freed from the anxiety which the painful feelings would have otherwise caused them, but in the process relationships with the (unknowing) recipient(s) of the projections become distorted (Segal, 1973; Klein, 1975). These processes can be applied to group functioning (Jaques, 1955; Menzies Lyth, 1960; Bion, 1961, etc.) whereby individuals in the same group

---

Box 2.3 Gerry's story continued.

Gerry was settled in his new flat and his care needs were being addressed. However he was having trouble. Throughout each day and night, he was spending periods of up to 3 hours at a time in the bathroom washing. No amount of coaxing or distraction could dissuade Gerry from this behaviour and his life was being severely curtailed through disruption of his sleep and difficulty in going out. Because of the psychological nature of this problem, it was decided to refer him to the clinical psychologist within the Community Mental Health Team.

Relationships between the social worker (the care coordinator) and the psychologist were cool. The social worker resented the higher status of the psychologist as well as his higher wage packet. She was envious of his ability to refuse to take on the care coordinator role within the team and thus avoid the responsibilities and tedious bureaucracy that this role entailed. On talking to her social work colleagues she found that they shared her feelings.

In turn, the psychologist distanced himself from the rest of the team. He set himself up in his own room, as had the doctors, leaving the majority of the team to work together in a noisy open-plan office. He was aware that his training was twice as long as the social worker's and in his heart felt that he was really a cut above her and deserved to be seen as the 'expert'. Unlike the social worker, his training had included no interprofessional education, the subject never arising, and he maintained strong allegiances to uni-professional working.

The social worker was reluctant to ask the psychologist for help in case it confirmed his position as expert and hers as unskilled general 'dogs body'. Their relationship was marked by a thinly veiled hostility and lack of cooperation. In the minds of both, a picture had been formed of their relationship that was informed by the realities of their different roles and training, yet also included a strong imaginary element which powerfully impacted on their joint work.

---

can share common anxieties and join forces with each other in projecting those difficult feelings onto another group. They thereby gain some relief from their anxieties while at the same time being enabled to identify with each other, thus strengthening their sense of group membership. As Hoggett (2004, p. 123) argues, 'in order to preserve its own identity each group tacitly manifests a desire to misunderstand the other'. We see then a collusion between the two groups, whereby in order for each to survive as a cohesive entity each must continue to act as the recipient of the other's projections.

Those who work in welfare services are tasked by their organisations and by society at large to work with and manage fundamental human difficulties such as illness, poverty and mental distress. In order to deal with the inevitable anxieties generated by the work, individuals, organised collectively in teams or subsystems, use systems of defence. It could be that the psychologist in the community team was aware that this was a privileged position as he was not expected to take the responsibilities of care coordination or 'get his hands dirty' with everyday concerns. He could have felt that other team members saw him as the expert who would be able to magically cure Gerry through the delivery of a few sessions of psychological help. This could have resulted in not only a sense of guilt but also a sense of failure resulting from the chronic and enduring nature of mental illness, a tide he could not stem, and the unrealistic expectation of the prevailing medical model which advocates 'treatment' and cure. This sense of failure and impotence may have been split off and located in the social worker who could thus have been seen by the psychologist as ineffective and inept. By sharing these projections with other members of his occupational group, the psychologist would have been able to strengthen his professional identity and sense of professional competence.

The social worker also operated defensive processes. She had worked with Gerry for over 6 years and had developed a good relationship with him. She visited him regularly and was emotionally affected by the difficulties and painful circumstances of his life. She had been involved in Gerry's compulsory admission to hospital and was in touch with the potential for further psychological disturbance. Her close encounter with this level of mental pain touched her own deep fears of 'madness', and in a team where supervision was the exception rather than the norm, she had little opportunity to think about and deal with these largely unconscious feelings. By splitting off and locating many of her bad feelings into another professional group, in this particular case this being the psychologists, the social worker could have gained some breathing space and ability to carry on. Just as with the psychologists, by sharing a collective process of splitting and projection with other social workers, their group identity would have been strengthened. Although this example relates to a social worker and clinical psychologist, this interprofessional acrimony could apply to any professional grouping.

So, to return to the idea of the relationship-in-the-mind, in addition to the real differences of each role is added a collection of imaginary differences emanating from the unconscious of each participant, and this is where significant problems in relating and working together exist. In order to facilitate a more effective working relationship, professionals need to openly acknowledge their imaginary differences. This of course requires a more reflexive awareness of the dynamics operating within teams and also the acceptance that interprofessional working can evoke emotional responses and that paying attention to these can be helpful and even necessary. Professionals need to be able to challenge their perceptions of others as well as rethink the way they see themselves.

Loxley (1997) acknowledges that conflict is inevitable within interprofessional working because each person brings with them a combination of social and professional differences, and this fuels the tendency to psychologically distance other groups. Stapleton (1998), for example, identifies significant differences in the per-spectives of physicians and midwives in the US as a factor that can create barriers and potential conflict. Each profession has its own culture comprising particular be-liefs, values and norms (see Chapter 1 for further discussion). Bion (1961) believed that every group, including professional groups, use particular psychological pro-cesses, or *basic assumptions* in their operation, each utilising different emotions and ideas in pursuit of their central task. Individuals are attracted to particular profes-sions for conscious and unconscious reasons. Where there is a psychological 'fit' with the particular emotions and values in operation within a certain profession, the individual, often unconsciously, would be drawn to that profession. This sug-gests that any differences between professional groups can be deeply personal and not easily overcome.

The different values and beliefs held by the professions lead them to construct their understanding of the nature of any problems and possible solutions to those problems in different ways (Stokes, 1994). Petrie (1976) uses the term *cognitive maps* to describe these different perspectives. A social worker may see the cause of mental distress as being rooted in structural inequalities in society, whereas a community psychiatric nurse could be more likely to accept the dominant 'medical model' and see the individual alone as responsible for their state of mind. In the former case, the social worker could see the best sort of help to offer would be in assisting the client to tackle social injustice, whereas the nurse may offer individual counselling or medication to address the problem. These different ways of seeing the world can cause severe clashes between professionals. As one social worker put it:

> It's hard ... it's two different perspectives coming to work together. They're bigger than us and they say 'why don't you just do what we ask?' We want to slow things down and look at it differently. So it's all this kind of underlying friction. (Keeping, 2006, p. 21)

Difference and potential conflict does not have to be problematic but can en-liven and stimulate practice if dealt with constructively, thereby facilitating a more holistic response to the needs of the service user. Teams who are always in agreement and engage in what Loxley (1997, p. 43) refers to as the *myth of togetherness* lose their potential for 'lateral and innovative thinking' (Hastings 2002, p. 117). How then can difference and conflict be viewed as a positive stimulus for change and creativity rather than something that should be avoided at all costs?

The key is honest communication within a safe environment where profes-sionals can explore one another's *cognitive maps* and where challenge and con-flict is accepted and dealt with openly. In order for this to happen, people need to be less defensive and keen to learn from each other. Professionals need to be supported to see conflict and difference in a positive light and recognise that when channelled appropriately it can act as a stimulus to creatively discuss ser-vice delivery (Barrett and Keeping, 2005). This, however, requires that conflict is acknowledged and openly discussed, a difficult but necessary task. In order to manage the inevitable anxiety this would create, there must be some way of containing it. The groups involved may be able to do so but more often than not; the containment needs to come from outside in the creation of a sufficiently robust and thoughtful environment where the principles of respect and safety predominate.

Power

A number of writers comment that in order to facilitate genuine participation and joint decision-making, relationships need to be recognised as interdependent and non-hierarchal in nature (Stapleton, 1998). This is no easy task as it requires an understanding and acceptance that within the interprofessional setting power is shared and fluctuates in accordance with whose knowledge and expertise best meets the needs of the client. Some may struggle with this as power has traditionally been sanctioned through authority and, within health and social care, has been located within the medical profession (Colyer, 2004). Hall (2005, p. 190) points out that doctors in Canada are 'trained to take charge and assume a role of leadership'. Relinquishing this traditionally based authority may be difficult for some as it may be perceived as a threat to professional role and identity.

In recent years, other occupational groups, traditionally considered to be semi-professions, have fought hard to gain recognition of their professional status, claiming autonomy based upon a distinct knowledge base and specialised sphere of practice. Sharing power can be perceived as a threat to professional autonomy and joint working can engender professional rivalry and envy if those involved feel that sharing erodes their status and unique position within health and social care practice.

In returning to our case study, it is easy to surmise that a significant factor at play in the relationship between the psychologist and the social worker was that of envy generated through status and pay differentials. In psychoanalytic terms envy is a very destructive force involving a mainly unconscious process whereby one individual psychologically attacks another who is perceived as having that which she/he desires (Klein, 1957/1975). Envy often emerges as a reaction to unbearable feelings of dependence upon someone and it thus has the potential to hurt not only the person under attack but also the attacker him/herself.

Although originally applied to intra- and interpersonal relationships, the concept of envy can be useful in understanding social systems (Stein, 2000). Many of the difficulties between different professional groups arise from competition for resources and power and, as Stokes (1994) notes, can closely resemble sibling rivalry. The endemic presence of envy within a social system can lead to malfunction and chaos. Stein identifies three ways in which envy can sabotage healthy functioning. Firstly, links with the envied 'other' can be broken so that all contact can be felt to be 'poisonous and malign'. It is thus not just the envied individual who is 'detested' (p. 204), but the very concept of any kind of link or association with that other person or group. Daum (2002) describes the difficulties the two teams he studied experienced in engaging in any joint venture, be it passing on a message or arranging and attending meetings together. He proposed that individuals were acting out their own feelings of envy by engaging in a collective unconscious envious attack on their colleagues (Daum, 2002, p. 130). The implications for interprofessional working are obvious.

Envy can also result in an attack on learning, given the feelings of dependence it can evoke. If, as Stein (2000) suggests, the very concept of learning engenders an undermining, envious attack, team members will lose the capacity to learn from each other, a necessary condition for interprofessional working.

The third way in which envy can sabotage group functioning is by engaging in an envious attack on authority figures. In interprofessional working, lines of power and accountability are often unclear, and conflicts based on envy can be focused on other members of the interprofessional team rather than on traditional authority figures.

An additional problem associated with the absence of clear lines of authority within a collaborative context is the potential to think that it is someone else's responsibility to implement agreed actions. Morrow et al. (2005) in a study of interprofessional working reported confusion regarding the issue of responsibility, and Allen et al. (2002) in researching health and social services provision in Wales identified a delay in the implementation of tasks when no one within the collaborative team took the lead. This is not always the case however and Abbott et al. (2005) reported on a subtle form of peer pressure which encouraged members of the interprofessional team to undertake the actions they had agreed to carry out.

An imbalance of power also has the potential to marginalise or oppress team members (Sullivan and Skelcher, 2002). Consequently, identifying the location of power is important and the following questions identified by Loxley (1997) can be used for this purpose: who defines power; whose terms are used; who controls the domain or territory; who decides upon what resources are needed and how they are allocated; who holds whom accountable; who prescribes the activity of others and who can influence policy makers?

Trust

In a paper drawing on evaluations of inter-agency networks in New Zealand, Walker (2004) identifies trust as being a central feature of all successful social relationships. In defining trust she stresses the importance of being able to rely upon another to behave in predictable ways. In the US, Mayer et al. (1995) propose a model of trust highlighting three key factors: confidence in the expertise and competence of the other; belief that others will behave altruistically rather than out of self-interest; and belief in the moral integrity of others. Within an interprofessional context, this relates to being able to depend upon respectful, honest and supportive relationships, which in turn are influenced by confidence, clarity of role and a secure sense of identity. Without trust, people may act defensively through, for example, withholding information, holding up progress by failing to attend meetings or being inflexible in their approach to cross-boundary working.

A sense of confidence is closely associated with self-image and perceptions of identity. Personal identity is developed early in life through a combination of innate constitutional factors and social relationships. There is a close link between personal and professional identity as it is likely that individuals will choose to join a particular profession as a way of expressing deeply held personal values and beliefs (Keeping, 2006). Once in place, the development of a clear professional role will also strengthen the sense of self. Professional identity develops through a process of socialisation which begins during initial education and develops through one's professional career. A positive professional identity is associated with professional competence and a clear understanding of one's role (Hornby and Atkins, 2000). Blurring of roles through overlap, duplication and flexible working can weaken professional identity, thus resulting in role insecurity and the potential for defensive responses, which can impede effective working relationships and sabotage the effective completion of task (Halton, 1994). It is thus important that each professional is clear about their own role in relation to that of their partners if interprofessional working is to be effective (Obholzer, 1994).

Roles are not always well defined (see Chapter 1 for further discussion of these issues). However, if a strong unifying characteristic is shared by others of the same professional group, this will serve to maintain a professional cohesiveness and a consequent sense of purpose and confidence. A study of social workers based in a team with other mental health professionals found that the role of social workers was ill-defined and varied from one worker to another (Keeping, 2006). However, all social workers adhered strongly to a common set of values which were seen as being central to their professional identity. In this case the maintenance of a secure professional identity was helped by having contact with other social work colleagues where the values underpinning the profession could be reinforced. In this way, the worker felt strengthened and less threatened by interprofessional working and more likely to cooperate and work with others. It is thus important that professionals are enabled to maintain links with their own professional group by the setting up of uni-professional supervision and meetings.

The lives of organisations cannot be understood without consideration of the social and political context in which they operate. Social relations are powerfully affected by political, economic and social circumstances, and thus relationships between organisational partners can be deeply affected by dynamics in operation within society. Particular difficulties within a society can be unconsciously acted out within institutions such as education, health and welfare, leading to falling productivity, an unhappy workforce and problematic relationships.

As an example, a study was undertaken within a school for black, physically disabled children in South Africa (Gibson and Swartz, 2001) at a time when South African society was struggling to come to terms with the impact of apartheid and the major social and political changes of recent years. A split had occurred within the staff group at the school between the teachers (who were both black and white) and the more junior crèche workers (all of whom were black), with the teachers accusing the junior workers of being lazy, uneducated and unkind to the children (incidentally, all terms once used by the powerful white minority against black people). There was very little contact between the groups, and a powerful fear of opening up unmanageable feelings prevented any useful dialogue between the two.

Consultants found that staff at the school were very reluctant to speak of the pain and difficulties experienced under the apartheid regime because of the profound feelings of loss and guilt lying just below the surface. They also found that people were very reluctant to discuss any kind of differences between people for fear that the deep divisions between black and white experienced under apartheid might be reactivated with all the fear and hatred this political system had evoked. Because of the reluctance to address the issue of difference, racial or otherwise, Gibson and Swartz suggest that staff were reluctant to talk openly with each other. The residue of painful feelings carried over from the time of apartheid, instead of being openly discussed and worked through, was instead being acted out within the staff group. The teachers thus projected their unwanted feelings onto the junior workers, thereby freeing themselves of these difficult feelings, and by sharing them with each other, promoted cohesion amongst their own group.

Clearly, the two staff groups needed to engage in open dialogue with each other in order to address those simmering resentments that both sides felt about the other. However, talking can only happen when people feel safe, and safety can be compromised by suspicion and the potential for misunderstanding. Gibson and Swartz suggest that secrecy and 'doublespeak' were the order of the day under apartheid and people have yet to trust that words can be trusted.

If interprofessional working is characterised by relationships dominated by the defensive processes of splitting and projection as identified earlier, the establishment of trust will be particularly difficult. It is only through open and honest communication in which those involved learn about and from each other that projections can be withdrawn and the process of trust can begin to grow. Trust therefore takes time to develop (Stapleton, 1998; Walker, 2004), is nurtured through respect and conveyed through the positive acknowledgement of one another's contribution to the interprofessional team. Time therefore needs to be devoted to enabling interprofessional team members to develop relationships, and to understand one another's *cognitive maps*, expert knowledge base and distinct role (see Box 2.4).

Box 2.4   Gerry's story continued.

The team manager was aware of the potential difficulties of collaborative working as she was in the process of undertaking a management course which addressed possible dilemmas in contemporary professional practice, including interprofessional working. She understood that professionals often need help in getting on with each other and that close working relationships can often evoke quite irrational emotional reactions. She had learnt that paying attention to these responses can be helpful and, indeed, necessary if the team is to function effectively.

Through a sensitive attunement to the emotional life of her team, she recognised that the social workers and psychologists appeared reluctant to engage with each other. While not wishing to pick on these two occupational groups, she decided to bring in an external facilitator to hold fortnightly supervision sessions where staff could bring any difficulties they were experiencing within the team. She felt that by supporting a culture of reflexive awareness she might encourage staff to be more open with each other about their inevitable differences. She recognised that this could be difficult and that the facilitator needed to be able to create a safe and supportive atmosphere in order to contain the anxieties of the group members.

Thus, it was that the social worker and psychologist were able to voice, at least, some of their feelings about the other. This wasn't easy as both found that in some ways it can be very satisfying to dislike another. Withdrawing these potentially damaging feelings involves a mental readjustment which requires psychological work and needs the individual to see himself or herself as well as the other in a new way.

The team manager at the same time realised that if the individual worker felt supported at work and happy and clear about their role, their sense of professional identity would be strengthened. She knew this would result in heightened confidence and a less defended staff member who would be less likely to envy and undermine the work of others. She thus supported each member of her team in accessing regular uni-professional meetings where they could gain the support of others from their own profession. She also ensured that each team member had access to regular caseload supervision and strove for an atmosphere whereby the very personal and difficult work of the team was acknowledged and respected.

Conclusion

From the above it can be seen that interprofessional working is not just a matter of contact and communication. Complex relational issues can facilitate or hinder collaborative practice. Interprofessional education has been identified as a means of enabling those involved to gain a better understanding of professional roles, challenge negative stereotypes and development effective communication (Barr *et al.*, 2000; Freeth *et al.*, 2002; Carpenter and Dickinson, 2008). However, interprofessional learning needs to encompass activities that enable those involved to develop a greater awareness of psychological defence mechanisms and facilitate the skills required to own up to feelings that may hinder collaboration and discuss these through open and honest communication. Learning experiences need to help professionals to value diversity, viewing it as a trigger that can enliven and stimulate debate, thus offering the potential for innovation and creativity.

Not all staff will have the opportunity to engage in formal educational experiences, and therefore informal learning opportunities within the workplace plus a combination of supervision and organisational/collegiate support all have a role to play in enabling those involved to set aside defences and engage collaboratively within the interprofessional arena.

Summary

- Despite the rhetoric calling for joined up thinking and action, interprofessional working has the potential to encounter many difficulties.
- Psychological dynamics have a significant part to play in the ability of groups of people to work interprofessionally.
- Social relations can evoke anxiety and result in the production of psychological defences which impede the task of collaborative working.
- These defensive processes are exacerbated by the distressing nature of the work involved in health and social care.
- Conflict needs to be acknowledged through a culture of reflexive awareness and openly discussed through honest communication in an environment where challenge is accepted and viewed positively as a stimulus for creativity and change.
- This process generates further anxiety that requires the provision of a robust and supportive environment generated through attention to group dynamics, supervision and an environment where trust, respect and safety predominate.

Further reading and relevant websites

Useful texts include:

Cooper, A. and Lousada, J. (2005) *Borderline Welfare: Feeling and Fear of Feeling in Modern Welfare*. London, Karnac.

Hornby, S. and Atkins, J. (2000) *Collaborative Care: Interprofessional, Interagency and Interpersonal*, 2nd edn. Oxford, Blackwell Science.

Loxley, A. (1997) *Collaboration in Health and Welfare: Working with Difference*. London, Jessica Kingsley Publishers.

Obholzer, A. and Zagier Roberts, V. (eds) *The Unconscious at Work: Individual and Organizational Stress in the Human Services*. London, Routledge.

Relevant websites include:

The Centre for the Advancement of Interprofessional Education is an independent UK charity working to promote more effective interprofessional education and learning: http://www.caipe.org.uk

The National Council for Voluntary Organisations Collaborative Working Unit offers practical advice and support for voluntary and community organisations considering whether and how to work collaboratively: http://www.ncvo-vol.org.uk/collaborativeworking-unit

The *Journal of Interprofessional Care* contains numerous articles on research, policy and practice related to interprofessional working: http://www.tandf.co.uk/journal/titles/13561820.html

References

Abbott, D., Townsley, R. and Watson, D. (2005) Multi-agency working in services for disabled children: what impact does it have on professionals? *Health and Social Care in the Community*, 13, 155–163.

Allen, D., Lyne, P. and Griffiths, L. (2002) Studying complex care interfaces: key issues arising from a study of multi-agency rehabilitative care for people who have suffered a stroke, *Journal of Clinical Nursing*, 11, 297–305.

Anderson, B. (1983) *Imagined Communities: Reflections on the Origins and Spread of Nationalism*. London, Verso.

Barr, H. *et al.* (2000) *Evaluations of Interprofessional Education: A United Kingdom Review for Health and Social Care*. London, Centre for the Advancement of Interprofessional Education/BERA.

Barrett, G. and Keeping, C. (2005) The processes required for effective interprofessional working, in G. Barrett, D. Sellman and J. Thomas (eds) *Interprofessional Working in Health and Social Care: Professional Perspectives*. Basingstoke, Palgrave Macmillan.

Bion, W.R. (1961) *Experiences in Groups*. London, Tavistock.

Carpenter, J. and Dickinson, H. (2008) *Interprofessional Education and Training*. Bristol, Policy Press.

Colyer, H.M. (2004) The construction and development of health professions: where will it end? *Journal of Advanced Nursing*, 48, 406–412.

Cooper, A. and Lousada, J. (2005) *Borderline Welfare: Feeling and Fear of Feeling in Modern Welfare*. London, Karnac.

Daum, M. (2002) Dangerous liaisons: projective identification, basic assumption envy, and the conflict between love and hate in the relationship between two psychiatric teams, *Organisational and Social Dynamics*, 2, 120–138.

Freeth, D. *et al.* (2002) *A Critical Review of Evaluations of Interprofessional Education*. Occasional Paper No. 2. London, Learning and Teaching Support Network for Health Sciences and Practice.

Gibson, K. and Swartz, L. (2001) Psychology, social transition and organizational life in South Africa: 'I can't change the past – but I can try', *Psychoanalytic Studies*, 3, 381–392.

Glasby, J. and Lester, H. (2004) Cases for change in mental health: partnership working in mental health services, *Journal of Interprofessional Care*, 18, 7–16.

Hall, P. (2005) Interprofessional teamwork: professional cultures as barriers, *Journal of Interprofessional Care*, 19(Suppl. 1), 188–196.

Halton, W. (1994) Some unconscious aspects of organizational life: contributions from psychoanalysis, in A. Obholzer and V. Zagier Roberts (eds) *The Unconscious at Work: Individual and Organizational Stress in the Human Services*. London, Routledge, pp. 11–19.

Hastings, M. (2002) Team working in rehabilitation, in A. Squires and M. Hastings (eds) *Rehabilitation of the Older Person*, 3rd edn. Cheltenham, Nelson Thornes, pp. 105–123.

Hoggett, P. (2004) Overcoming the desire for misunderstanding through dialogue, in S. Snape. and P. Taylor (eds) *Partnerships between Health and Local Government*. London, Frank Cass & Co., pp. 118–128.

Hornby, S. and Atkins, J. (2000) *Collaborative Care: Interprofessional, Interagency and Interpersonal*, 2nd edn. Oxford, Blackwell Science.

Hudson, B. and Henwood, M. (2002) The NHS and social care: the final countdown, *Policy and Politics*, 30, 153–166.

Jaques, E. (1955) The social system as a defence against persecutory and depressive anxiety, in M. Klein, P. Heimann and R. Money-Kyrle (eds) *New Directions in Psychoanalysis*. Tavistock, London, pp. 478–498.

Keeping, C. (2006) *Emotional Aspects of the Professional Identity of Social Workers: A Study of Social Workers Working with Avon and Wiltshire Mental Health Partnership NHS Trust*. Bristol, University of the West of England and Avon and Wiltshire Mental Health Partnership NHS Trust.

Klein, M. (1957/1975) *Envy and Gratitude and Other Works 1946–1963*. London, Hogarth Press.

Klein, M. (1975) *The Writings of Melanie Klein*, Vol. 3. London, Hogarth Press.

Loxley, A. (1997) *Collaboration in Health and Welfare: Working with Difference*. London, Jessica Kingsley Publishers.

Mayer, R., Davies, J.H. and Schoorman, F.D. (1995) An integrative model of organizational trust, *Academy of Management Review*, 20, 709–734.

Menzies Lyth, I. (1960) *Containing Anxiety in Institutions* (1988). London, Free Association Books.

Morrow, G., Malin, N. and Jennings, T. (2005) Interprofessional teamworking for child and family referral in a Sure Start local programme, *Journal of Interprofessional Care*, 19, 93–101.

Obholzer, A. (1994) Authority, power and leadership: contributions from group relations training, in A. Obholzer and V. Zagier Roberts (eds) *The Unconscious at Work: Individual and Organizational Stress in the Human Services*. London, Routledge, pp. 39–47.

Petrie, H. (1976) Do you see what I see? The epistemology of interdisciplinary inquiry, *Journal of Aesthetic Education*, 10, 29–43.

Segal, H. (1973) *Introduction to the Work of Melanie Klein*. London, Hogarth Press.

Simmel, G. (1955) *Conflict and the Web of Group-Affiliations* (Translated from German by K.H. Wolff and R. Bendix). London, Collier-Macmillan.

Stapleton, S.R. (1998) Team-building: making collaborative practice work, *Journal of Nursing and Midwifery*, 43, 12–18.

Stein, M. (2000) After Eden: envy and the defences against anxiety paradigm, *Human Relations*, 53, 193–211.

Stokes, J. (1994) Institutional chaos and personal stress, in A. Obholzer and V. Zagier Roberts (eds) *The Unconscious at Work: Individual and Organizational Stress in the Human Services.* London, Routledge, pp. 121–128.

Sullivan, H. and Skelcher, C. (2002) *Working across Boundaries: Collaboration in Public Services.* Basingstoke, Palgrave.

Walker, A. (2004) *Overcoming the Neo-liberal Legacy: The Importance of Trust for Improved Interagency Collaborative Working in New Zealand.* Research Paper No. 11. Auckland, Local Partnerships and Governance Research Group, University of Auckland.

3 Partnership working: key concepts and approaches

Walter Leutz

Building on previous discussions of culture and of interprofessional practice, aims this chapter to propose useful concepts for thinking about current approaches to partnership working and service integration. My thinking is based on more than 25 years as a developer, evaluator and academic observer of efforts to integrate acute care, long-term care (LTC) and other support services designed for individuals with disabilities. This includes development and evaluation of US Social Health Maintenance Organisations (HMOs), which since 1985 have offered a benefit that integrates Medicare acute care services with privately financed community care benefits in a managed care model (Leutz *et al.*, 1985, 1991; Fischer *et al.*, 1998). I also helped the Kaiser Permanente HMO develop a demonstration of how to connect with community-based LTC services for its members with disabilities (Leutz *et al.*, 2003a, b). More recently I was part of a team that evaluated 11 demonstration programmes in three states that have integrated Medicare acute care and Medicaid LTC in managed care models for individuals dually eligible for both programmes (Bishop *et al.*, 2007; Leutz *et al.*, 2007). More details on these and other US integration initiatives are covered by Dennis Kodner in Chapter 5 (see also Box 3.1 for a brief summary of key US terms and acronyms).

The public purchase of integrated, privately managed care in the Social HMO, dual-eligible programmes and similar initiatives shows that the new public management tenet of privatisation (see Introduction for further discussion) has been linked with US integration initiatives for more than 20 years. Beginning with On Lok/PACE (Branch *et al.*, 1995) and Social HMOs in the mid-1980s, and then with the Medicare/Medicaid integration initiative that spurred dual-eligible demonstrations in the 1990s (George Mason University, 2007), integration seemed destined to be incorporated into the mainline Medicare and Medicaid programmes through legislation and bureaucratic support. First, PACE was made permanent and Social HMOs were extended in the Balanced Budget Act of 1997; and then – with the backing of Social HMOs, dual-eligible plans and EverCare (which provides managed acute care services to nursing facility residents) – a new type of Medicare managed care plan (the Special Needs Plan or SNP) was created in the Medicare Modernization Act of 2003 (Achman and Harris, 2005).

Box 3.1 US terms and acronyms.

- *Dual eligibles*. Individuals who are eligible for both Medicare and Medicaid.
- *EverCare*. An HMO that enrols nursing home residents, developed first as a demonstration but now available for other managed care organisations.
- *HMO (Health Maintenance Organisation)*. A private managed care organisation that owns or contracts for the full range of acute care services and delivers them to enrolled members.
- *Medicaid*. The public insurance programme for the poor, operated by states and funded jointly by federal and state general revenues. It covers acute care and long-term care.
- *Medicare*. The public insurance programme for acute care for retirees and the disabled, funded by payroll taxes and general revenues.
- *Medicare Advantage*. The approach to Medicare HMOs legislated in 2003.
- *PACE* (The Program for All-Inclusive Care for the Elderly, an HMO for very disabled elders who are eligible for both Medicare and Medicaid and who reside in the community. Started as the On Lok demonstration) and made permanent in 1997.
- *Social HMO*. A Medicare HMO demonstration that adds a community-based long-term care benefit to standard Medicare services.
- *SNP (Special Needs Plan)*. A Medicare HMO that enrols individuals who have specified chronic illnesses or disabilities, who reside in nursing homes or who are eligible for Medicaid.

Unfortunately, the regulations that have been developed so far to implement SNPs do not require them to do much that is 'special': they do not have any requirements for integration, but they also introduce some new barriers to integration. I will return to the details of these new developments in the Discussion section. First, I will review the 'laws' of integration and how they can be used.

Using the 'laws of integration'

This section builds on my previously published thoughts on 'laws of integration' – five in the original article (Leutz, 1999) and four more on reflection (Leutz, 2005) (see Box 3.2). The laws are based on analyses of integration efforts in the US and the UK, mostly in the 1990s, and were developed with particular reference to services for frail and disabled people. The question that spurred this thinking was a simple one raised by Bleddyn Davies, who was my mentor during a sabbatical in the UK in 1997. He kept asking, who really needs the extensively integrated services and financing of the PACE model? I ended up turning the question on its head by asking, who needs other kinds and levels of integration? The result was a framework for thinking about how to design joint working according to the needs

---

Box 3.2   Laws of integration (original five plus four on reflection).

1. You can integrate some of the services for all of the people, or all of the services for some of the people, but you can't integrate all the services for all the people.
2. Integration costs before it pays.
3. Your integration is my fragmentation.
4. You can't integrate a square peg and a round hole.
5. The one who integrates calls the tune.
6. All integration is local.
7. Keep it simple, stupid.
8. Don't try to integrate everything.
9. Integration isn't built in a day.

---

of the populations served. This framework will be discussed in the first section below. This will be followed by a discussion of key challenges to creating and maintaining integrated services and then a review of a few practical guides to designing integration initiatives.

A framework

The first 'law', which paraphrases Abraham Lincoln's comment about fooling the people, provides a portal for thinking about the design of integration initiatives. It first focuses on what kind of acute and social support services people with disabilities need, and in turn, on what services might be integrated to meet those needs. The original article identified three prototype levels of integration: full integration, coordination and linkage. 'Full integration' is at the 'all of the services for some of the people' end of the spectrum and is appropriate for those who are very dependent in LTC and perhaps unstable medically. A good example of full integration is PACE, which serves a nursing home eligible community-dwelling population. It operates with pooled financing for all acute and LTC benefits, team care management, supportive housing and more (Chatterji et al., 1998).

At the other end of integration is 'linkage' ('some of the services for all of the people'). In a system with linkage, populations are screened to identify emergent LTC needs; clinicians in various settings understand and respond to the needs of persons with disabilities; and people with needs are provided with accurate information about services and assistance with access if needed through referrals. Linkage may be all that is needed for those who can self-manage. To qualify as an integration effort, linkage mechanisms need to be present in acute care settings, since that is where new LTC needs often emerge.

A good example of a linkage initiative is a demonstration that the Kaiser Permanente HMO initiated in 1995 to show how to expand its scope of services to include a broad range of home- and community-based services that would be easily accessible to people with functional disabilities (Leutz *et al.*, 2003a, b). The most common feature of linkage models proposed and tested by practitioners from the Kaiser Permanente system was a person designated as a 'single point of contact' (SPOC). The SPOC worked first with community providers to understand their services and how to make effective referrals (e.g. get the prospective client to sign a release so that the community provider could contact them), and then with medical system clinicians to help them identify patients who might benefit and to make a simple referral to the SPOC, who took over making connections.

The middle level of integration is 'coordination', which is appropriate for the varied 'some of the services for some of the people' group not explicitly mentioned in the first law. The hallmark of coordination is care management of individuals using acute and LTC services sequentially or simultaneously. This level of assistance is appropriate for individuals with extensive and complex needs who have strong informal support, or for individuals with more moderate needs who have weak informal support.

The care coordination function of US Social HMOs is a good example of coordination. For example, care managers work with hospital discharge planners and home health nurses to help manage transitions from medical care to LTC benefits and services; most sites have ways to access medical records and include LTC services in medical charts, and all created LTC benefits and services to fill gaps in medical coverage (Abrahams *et al.*, 1992a, b). An example of the latter was inclusion of bathroom safety devices in LTC benefits to fill a glaring gap in Medicare benefits ('Medicare stops at the bathroom door' is the tag line in the field). One site paid for the equipment and installation with the LTC benefit and then used the Medicare home health benefit to bring in staff to train beneficiaries in their use (Leutz *et al.*, 2005; Leutz and Capitman, 2007).

The original article laid out how these three levels of integration differed on what they did regarding population screening, clinical practice, transitions and service delivery, information sharing, case management, benefits, and the dimensions and severity of service user needs they were able to address. The second article highlighted the fact that real world integration programmes may be fully integrated in some dimensions and coordinated or even linked in others.

One example of this is Social HMOs, which integrate financing but at best coordinate rather than integrate service delivery. Even the Social HMO II site, which was designed to be more integrated with medical care than the original sites, kept its medical care screening and care coordination team separate from its LTC benefit screening and care coordination team (Leutz and Capitman, 2007). Similarly, all of the dual demonstration models receive capitated payments for a full range of acute and LTC services, but only the Wisconsin Partnership sites are fully integrated through a multidisciplinary team for care management (Malone *et al.*, 2004; Bishop *et al.*, 2007). In contrast, the Minnesota and Massachusetts models coordinate through care managers, similar to Social HMOs. The Wisconsin Partnership Program (2007) chose to go further in care coordination because its model enrols only the most at risk, while the other two enrol the full spectrum of the Medicare/Medicaid population (Minnesota Senior Health Options, 2007).

The second article also emphasised the idea that more integration is not necessarily better and posed the law of 'keep it simple, stupid' (the advice Bill Clinton's campaign staff gave him in the 1992 presidential race). An example of a simple system of integration is found in the Japanese LTC insurance system, which is separately financed and operated from medical care. However, the designers, in order to save money on acute care insurance, moved skilled home health into the LTC benefit. A small pilot study of LTC insurance care coordination found that these nurses had two-way communication and coordination with nurses in primary care offices concerning monitoring of complex conditions, therapies and discharge planning (Leutz and Ikegami, 2004). Another reason not to integrate more than is needed, especially in the area of pooled finances, is the danger of 'upward substitution' of pooled resources into the more powerful acute care system. Linkage and coordination models can be designed explicitly to strengthen the weaker community care partner in integration schemes.

Finally, in terms of Glasby and Dickinson's introduction to this book, it is worth emphasising that it does not do a lot of good to be integrated at the organisational and structural levels if you are not integrated at the client/individual/service delivery level. That is, do inter-organisational agreements actually get clinicians and care managers to work together in new ways? Conversely, if front-line staff have already figured out ways to be integrated at the individual level, it may not be necessary to go to the trouble of integrating at the broader levels. This more informal approach to integration may work better for linkage than coordination, since it is the higher levels of organisations and systems that tend to have the resources necessary to pay for coordination's care management, information systems and new benefits.

The challenges of integration

As the foregoing discussion shows, developing and maintaining joint working is a challenge. Several of the original and new laws speak to the reasons for this, but the fourth – you can't integrate a square peg in a round hole – may be most important. The fourth law speaks both to the different, if not conflicting, cultures of acute and LTC (see Chapter 1) and to the fact that health and social care systems are set up separately from the top (legislative committees), through the middles (bureaucracies and provider organisations), to the bottom (professionals and other direct care personnel). The same could be said about differences with other service systems and cultures (e.g. mental health, housing and intellectual disabilities). Acute care and LTC differ in multiple dimensions, including the following:

- *Clinical orientation.* Diagnose and cure disease in acute care versus assess functional status and address deficits in LTC.
- *Financing.* Universal entitlements versus means-tested programmes.
- *Administration.* National versus state and local.
- *Provider organisations.* Hospitals and rehabilitation facilities versus community care agencies and residential facilities.

- *Staff*. Physicians and nurses versus social workers, paraprofessionals and families.
- *Access*. Relatively smooth through doctors' orders versus diverse systems with caps and waits and exclusions.
- *Benefits*. A relatively uniform core versus geographic differences in coverage and availability.

For most professionals, managers, bureaucrats and legislators, the day-to-day reality of getting the job done is more about within-system matters than cross-systems matters. Working effectively with the other side requires time, learning, change, sharing, compromise, and bending or re-writing rules and protocols. Time, entropy and turnover tend to pull innovations and innovators back to standard within-sector practice.

Guides to integration

Lessons from past attempts at joint working can be tapped to provide additional guides for future efforts. One lesson embodied in the original laws – integration costs before it pays – is that it is important to put new resources into the mix rather than planning for savings from the outset. If the acute and LTC partners to integration are expected to use their current resources to do new jobs or the other side's job, they are likely to balk, since they have more than enough to do already. Alternatively, new resources can help both sides to address common challenges from a win-win perspective.

A second guide is that it is usually best to empower social care to take the lead in designing and operating joint ventures. Social care is often the weaker partner, and this power imbalance can make it fearful of potential dominance by the acute sector. Another original law states that 'the one who integrates calls the tune'. The tune of social care providers is more likely to be integration, whereas medical providers are more likely to define the problem and the needs in medical terms. This was seen in early UK efforts to integrate, which gave physicians in total purchasing pilot fundholding practices the responsibility to design integration with community care – perhaps unsurprisingly, they tended to prioritise their own services (Mays, 1997; Myles *et al.*, 1997).

Notwithstanding this advice, a third guide is that it is imperative that would-be integrators understand the demands that integration places on medical care providers and that they do not make new demands that cannot be met. Another original law – your integration is my fragmentation – speaks to this point primarily from the perspective of busy physicians. There are many, many demands for physicians to add just one more small thing to their routines to address a very wide range of clinical care and public health needs. If integration initiatives add just one small thing for physicians to do for each of the numerous LTC populations, doctors will likely experience these integration attempts as fragmentation and resist.

An alternative is to ask for something very small and to offer in return something that will make the physician's life easier. The Kaiser Permanente demonstration had a good example of this in its dementia model of care. A pilot study found that primary care physicians and even neurologists were hesitant to diagnose dementia because they did not want to give families such devastating news when the medical system had nothing to offer. After the demonstration set up a referral relationship with the Alzheimer's Association and physicians were trained to make an internal referral to a single point of contact, diagnoses rose, in part because physicians said they had something to offer (Leutz et al., 2003b).

A fourth guide is to be flexible about integration requirements. This is in part related to another law added later – all integration is local. On the one hand, local practitioners and agencies develop informal ways to coordinate care even in the absence of official programmes (see, e.g., Foote and Stanners, 2002). One would not want to undo useful instances of this. On the other hand, official programmes should be cognisant of the fact that care problems and the potential for solutions differ by community. If local professionals, organisations and citizens are given the freedom and responsibility to define problems, solutions and pace within a broad framework, they may be more likely to engage than they are in top-down initiatives.

Fifth, it is imperative for efforts at joint working to figure out how to ac-commodate choice/autonomy/control by service users. In the US, advocates of consumer-directed LTC models tend to contrast consumer direction to control of services by professionals, and to tout the advantages of choosing and managing one's own services over being a passive patient in a 'medical model' of care (Batavia et al., 1991). This thinking is compelling but not very accommodating for integration initiatives, which tend to rely on case managers and professional teams (Leutz, 1998). One way to bridge this gap may be to extend integration to include service users and caregivers using Harvath and colleagues' concept of 'local and cosmopolitan knowledge' (Harvath et al., 1994). In LTC, the family brings local knowledge of service user preferences and capabilities, and the professional (in their model, the nurse) brings cosmopolitan knowledge of health conditions and service systems. Harvath and colleagues recommend four approaches to working through coordination with service users and carers: recognise the local when it works; enhance the local when it does not; help families apply local knowledge to problem solving; and blend local and cosmopolitan knowledge. Duffy and O'Brien provide additional perspectives on consumer-directed care in Chapter 10.

Finally, it is important that any evaluation of joint working is tailored to the objectives and mechanisms of the specific initiative. One of the most damaging evaluation findings regarding the Social HMOs was that they failed to integrate acute and social care (Harrington et al., 1993). This conclusion was based on the fact that physicians had not been included on the case management team and often did not even know that their patients were receiving Social HMO LTC benefits. The demonstration sites responded that the evaluators were imposing their own model of clinical integration (full integration) rather than evaluating the model that sites had developed (coordination) (Leutz, 1995). That is, the sites were not attempting to include physicians in a fully integrated system but were rather trying to coordinate care through work with hospital discharge planners, home health nurses and access to medical records. A good example of well-targeted research on joint working is found in the evaluation of the implementation and impact of PRISMA (Hébert *et al.*, 2005; Hébert and Veil, 2005; see also Chapters 5 and 11). The evaluation team first worked with project staff to define the components of the intervention and their relative importance; then had them assess the degree to which they were implemented; and then assessed impacts in the light of the degree of implementation at different test sites.

Discussion

Much has been learned from more than two decades of integration initiatives in the US, and many of these lessons may well be applicable in other systems. Despite this, the heyday of integration as a hope for solving cost and quality problems in US acute care and LTC may be over. Backers of the Special Needs Plan (SNP) provisions of the 2003 Medicare Modernization Act had hoped that the law would provide a permanent home to Social HMOs, dual-eligible plans and other demonstration integration initiatives, but the new requirements for Medicare Advantage plans (the new name for Medicare HMOs), as well as regulations for SNPs, are not supportive of integration. The specific Medicare programme alterations that made integration possible in demonstrations have been stripped away.

Firstly, Medicare Advantage plans (SNPs included) must now account for and report in much more detail how Medicare funds are spent. Savings (the difference between Medicare revenues and expenses for Medicare services – now called a 'rebate') – can be spent only on approved supplements, and LTC services (e.g. personal care and homemakers) are explicitly excluded. Secondly, there is no place in Medicare's information website for Social HMOs and dual-eligible programmes to list their LTC and care coordination benefits. Thus, even if an SNP or other Medicare Advantage programme wanted to market an LTC supplement in conjunction with a Medicare plan, they would be disadvantaged advertising for it. Thirdly, the only difference between the SNP regulations and the regular Medicare Advantage plans is to allow SNPs to enrol 'Special Needs' subgroups of the Medicare population (i.e. those with serious chronic illnesses and disabilities, dual eligibles and those residing in nursing facilities). The latter category incorporated the EverCare model, but EverCare has never been a true integration initiative, since EverCare manages only medical and acute care services and does not alter the delivery of nursing home care (Kane *et al.*, 2002). For SNPs serving special needs beneficiaries in the community (the category of SNPs designed for Social HMOs and dual-eligible plans), so far there are no requirements for these Medicare plans to coordinate payment and service delivery with Medicaid LTC services or to offer any special benefits or services.

Fourthly, the Medicare disability-based payment system that has sustained Social HMOs and dual-eligible plans against adverse selection (Kautter and Pope, 2005; Leutz *et al.*, 2007b) is not being offered to new SNPs and will be phased out for Social

HMOs and dual-eligible plans between 2008 and 2010. These provisions essentially disassemble Social HMOs, since these plans will no longer be able to finance LTC through Medicare savings, market their integrated services or be protected against adverse selection on disability. The Centers for Medicare and Medicaid Services have given the four operating sites two options for phasing down between 2008 and 2010: (1) continue financing and offering LTC for 3 years, but close the plan to new enrolment as of January 2008, or (2) keep enrolment open but eliminate LTC benefits. Two Social HMO sites – SCAN and Kaiser Permanente – took the former option, while two – Elderplan and Sierra – took the latter.

The dual-eligible demonstrations face the same phase down of disability-based payment, but they are advantaged compared to Social HMOs in that Medicaid pays for their LTC benefits (i.e. they do not need to finance these benefits from Medicare savings). However, our recent evaluation of the effect of the Medicare Modernization Act on dual demos was that extensive new requirements for tracking and reporting on spending on Medicare services may be leading to 'disintegration on paper' and 'cost-ineffective' care (Leutz et al., 2007a).

On the Medicaid side, attention has turned to integrating Medicaid LTC services under the banner of consumer choice, spurred by a 1999 Supreme Court decision to redress inequities in access to Medicaid-funded LTC services (Rosenbaum, 2000). The federal government undertook a series of 'systems change' initiatives (Walsh et al., 2006) – for example, Money Follows the Person (Anderson et al., 2006), in Medicaid, which seeks to integrate LTC decision-making and give service users more say. Integration with acute care services has not been a goal of these initiatives.

In summary, except for making PACE permanent in the 1997 Balanced Budget Act, the US Congress has not included mechanisms for acute/LTC integration in new policies for Medicare or Medicaid. In fact, the policy foundation for integration has become less friendly as specific supports (funds pooling to support care coordination and expanded benefits, disability-based reimbursement, etc.) have been withdrawn. This has undermined existing integration initiatives and discouraged new ones. At the broadest level of metaphor, Congress has re-rounded the hole that the square integration peg had been trying to carve out.

In retrospect, it is not clear that there has ever been broad policy support for integration as a serious strategy to reform US health care. The initiative for integration came primarily from the private provider side (including some HMOs but more strongly from LTC providers) and from a few states. When initial evaluations of Social HMOs were negative (Manton et al., 1993; Newcomer, 1993; Newcomer et al., 1995, 1996) but disputed (Leutz and Greenlick, 1995, 1998) and evaluations of dual-eligible plans were mixed (Kane and Homyak, 2003, 2004), many policy makers lost enthusiasm for integration as a means to control costs and improve outcomes. Mainstream policy makers in Congress, states and the bureaucracy had been willing to give reformers the chance to demonstrate their models, but they were not willing to stick with and refine models, or to try new approaches, when initial trials could not demonstrate conclusively better results. Although PACE was made permanent in the 1997 Balanced Budget Act, other provisions of the Act, as well as the 2003 Medicare Modernization Act, reverted to the traditional approach of dealing with acute care Medicare separately from LTC.

In summary, support in the US for integrating acute care and LTC has never been broad enough or deep enough to sustain lasting change. Perhaps this is not surprising, given the retreat from health planning and the turn to market-based systems more than 20 years ago. Integration was relegated to the province of managed care programmes, which in most states have never enrolled more than a small fraction of the Medicare and Medicaid populations. The mainstream fee-for-service payment system remained focused entirely on the delivery of discrete services or episodes of service. Coordination with LTC, particularly community-based LTC, has never been a requirement. Moreover, participation in integration has always been optional – for provider sponsors of integrated managed care programmes and even for states (e.g. PACE and the dual-eligible initiatives are state options). There have never been any requirements for regular Medicare HMOs to do anything to coordinate care with non-Medicare LTC programmes. Serious efforts to create joint working in the US will require a return of a willingness to acknowledge the problems of a fragmented approach, a readiness to develop strong policy initiatives to compel public programmes and private providers to participate, and a willingness to stick with initiatives until results are achieved. While this chapter has focused on US case studies, other chapters suggest that the same could also be true of other health and social care systems internationally. In particular, the US experience might suggest a tenth law that could be just as applicable to other systems – *don't put all your integration in one basket*. That is, if one of the partners in integration (in this case, Medicare policy makers) gets cold feet, you had better have another.

Summary

- There is a broad range of types and levels of disability and chronic illness in the population, which are associated with different and changing needs for acute care and LTC services.
- Initiatives for joint working should be designed to integrate in different ways and to different degrees to meet diverse needs.
- An inherent barrier to integration is the fact that acute and LTC occupy different policy and practice universes, in terms of clinical orientation, financing, administration, provider organisations, staff, accessibility and benefits.
- Joint working requires upfront investments to build systems and to win cooperation from collaborating agencies and practitioners.
- Because social care is typically the advocate for integration, but also the weaker partner in terms of power and service resources, it may be advisable to empower them through joint working structures.
- Physicians are more likely to cooperate in joint working if demands on them are minimised and also repaid by helping them solve problems posed by their patients with disabilities.

- Top-down models for joint working should allow for local flexibility and innovation.
- Professionally driven integration initiatives can find ways to respect, rely on and strengthen the preferences of service users and carers, while offering them the value of knowledge and system connections.
- Evaluations of joint working should focus on what programmes actually do, rather than on what evaluators think they should be doing.
- Aside from PACE, long-standing US integration initiatives are being dismantled by changes in federal policy that seek improvements in acute care and LTC efficiency and outcomes separately rather than jointly.

Further reading and relevant websites

For the earlier discussions of the 'laws of integration', see:
Leutz, W. (1999) Five laws for integrating medical and social care: lessons from the US and UK, *Milbank Quarterly*, 77(1), 77–110.
Leutz, W. (2005) Reflections on integrating medical and social care: five laws revisited, *Journal of Integrated Care*, 13(5), 3–12.

For examples of how Social HMOs coordinate social and medical care, see:
Abrahams, R. *et al.* (1992a) Across the great divide: integrating acute, post-acute, and long-term care, *Journal of Case Management*, 1(4), 124–134.
Leutz, W. and Greenlick, M. (1998) *The Social HMO Demonstration: Myths and Realities Reconsidered*. Available online via http://socialhmo.brandeis.edu/

For detailed discussions and examples of how state dual-eligible initiatives coordinate social and medical care, see:
Bishop, C. *et al.* (2007) *Medicare Special Needs Plans: Lessons from Dual-Eligible Demonstrations for CMS, States, Health Plans and Providers*. Report to CMS under Task Order Proposal (RTOP) No. CMS-04-016/VAC. Waltham, MA, Brandeis University (see CMS web link below).
Malone, J. *et al.* (2004) *MSHO Care Coordination Study: Final Report*. St Paul, Minnesota Department of Human Services (see state web link below).

For a detailed narrative of the development of a local UK integration initiative, see:
Foote, C. and Stanners, C. (2002) *Integrating Care for Older People*. London, Jessica Kingsley.

A wide range of international articles and reviews of integration can be found in the *International Journal of Integrated Care*: http://www.ijic.org

Information on the PACE programme can be found on two websites:
The National PACE association website explains the model and recent developments: http://www.npaonline.org/website/
The Medicare website contains updates and evaluation studies: http://www.medicare.gov/Nursing/Alternatives/Pace.asp

Data and studies concerning the Minnesota Senior Health Options (MSHO) dual-eligible demonstration are found on the State government website:
http://www.dhs.state.mn.us/main/idcplg?IdcService = GET_DYNAMIC_CONVERSION

Data and studies concerning the Wisconsin Partnership Program dual-eligible demonstration are found on the State government website:
http://dhfs.wisconsin.gov/wipartnership/

Data and studies concerning the Social HMO can be found on the Brandeis University website: http://socialhmo.brandeis.edu/

The Centers for Medicare and Medicaid Services website provides online access to a wide range of evaluations of demonstration projects:
For Medicare projects, see
http://www.cms.hhs.gov/DemoProjectsEvalRpts/MD/list.asp#TopOfPage
For Medicaid projects, see
http://www.cms.hhs.gov/demoprojectsevalrpts/EMD/list.asp#topofpage

References

Abrahams, R. *et al.* (1992a) Across the great divide: integrating acute, post-acute, and long-term care, *Journal of Case Management*, 1(4), 124–134.

Abrahams, R. *et al.* (1992b) Integrating care for the geriatric patient: examples from the Social HMO, *HMO Practice*, 6(4), 14–19.

Achman, L. and Harris, L. (2005) *Early Effects of the Medicare Modernization Act: Benefits, Cost Sharing, and Premiums of MA Plans, 2005.* Washington, DC, AARP Public Policy Institute.

Anderson, W. *et al.* (2006) *Money Follows the Person Initiatives of the Systems Change Grantees.* Report from RTI International to the Centers for Medicare and Medicaid Services, Baltimore, MD.

Batavia, A. *et al.* (1991) Toward a national personal assistance program: the independent living model of long-term care for persons with disabilities, *Journal of Health Politics, Policy and Law*, 16(3), 523–545.

Bishop, C. *et al.* (2007) *Medicare Special Needs Plans: Lessons from Dual-Eligible Demonstrations for CMS, States, Health Plans, and Providers*, Report to CMS under Task Order Proposal (RTOP) No. CMS-04–016/VAC. Waltham, MA, Brandeis University.

Branch, L. *et al.* (1995) The PACE evaluation: initial findings, *Gerontologist*, 35(3), 349–359.

Chatterji, P. *et al.* (1998) *Evaluation of the PACE Demonstration: The Impact of PACE on Participant Outcomes.* Cambridge, MA, Abt Associates.

Fischer, L. *et al.* (1998) The closing of a Social HMO: a case study, *Journal of Aging and Social Policy*, 10(1), 57–76.

Foote, C. and Stanners, C. (2002) *Integrating Care for Older People.* London, Jessica Kingsley.

George Mason University (2007) *Medicare Medicaid Integration Program.* Fairfax, VA, George Mason University. Available online via http://www.gmu.edu/departments/chpre/research/MMIP/.

Harrington, C. *et al.* (1993) Medical services in social health maintenance organizations, *Gerontologist*, 33(6), 790–800.

Harvath, T. *et al.* (1994) Establishing partnerships with family caregivers: local and cosmopolitan knowledge, *Journal of Gerontological Nursing*, 20(2), 29–35.

Hébert, R., Tourigny, A. and Gagnon, M. (2005) *Integrated Service Delivery to Ensure Persons' Functional Autonomy*. Montreal, EDISEM.

Hébert, R. and Veil, A. (2005) Monitoring the degree of implementation of an integrated delivery system, *International Journal of Integrated Care*, 5. Available online via http://www.ijic.org

Kane, R. *et al.* (2002) *Evaluation of the EverCare Demonstration Program*. Minneapolis, University of Minnesota.

Kane, R. and Homyak, P. (2003) *Multi State Evaluation of Dual Eligibles Demonstration: Minnesota Senior Health Options Evaluation*. Minneapolis, University of Minnesota.

Kane, R. and Homyak, P. (2004) *Multi State Evaluation of Dual Eligibles Demonstration: Wisconsin Partnership Program Evaluation*. Minneapolis, University of Minnesota.

Kautter, J. and Pope, G.C. (2005) CMS frailty adjustment model, *Health Care Finance Review*, 26(2), 1–19.

Leutz, W. (1995) Medical services in Social HMOs: a reply to Harrington *et al.*, *The Gerontologist*, 35(1), 6–8.

Leutz, W. (1998) Home care benefits for persons with disabilities, *American Rehabilitation*, 24(3), 6–14.

Leutz, W. (1999) Five laws for integrating medical and social care: lessons from the US and UK, *Milbank Quarterly*, 77(1), 77–110.

Leutz, W. (2005) Reflections on integrating medical and social care: five laws revisited, *Journal of Integrated Care*, 13(5), 3–12.

Leutz, W. and Capitman, J. (2007) Met needs, unmet needs, and satisfaction among Social HMO members, *Journal of Aging and Social Policy*, 19(1), 1–20.

Leutz, W. *et al.* (1985) *Changing Health Care for an Aging Society: Planning for the Social Health Maintenance Organization*. Lexington, MA, Lexington Books.

Leutz, W. *et al.* (1991) Adding long-term care to medicare in HMOs: four years of Social HMO experience, *Journal of Aging and Social Policy*, 4(3), 69–88.

Leutz, W. *et al.* (2003a) *Linking Medical Care and Community Services: Practical Models for Bridging the Gap*. New York, Springer.

Leutz, W. *et al.* (2003b) Kaiser Permanente's manifesto 2005 demonstration: the promises and limits of devolution, *Journal of Aging and Social Policy*, 14(3–4), 233–244.

Leutz, W. *et al.* (2005) Utilization and costs of home-based and community-based care within a Social HMO: trends over an 18 year period, *International Journal of Integrated Care*. Available online via http://www.ijic.org

Leutz, W. *et al.* (2007a) *Examination of the Changing Context for Dual Demonstration Contractors*. Report to CMS under Task Order Proposal (RTOP) No CMS-04–016/VAC. Waltham, MA, Brandeis University.

Leutz, W. *et al.* (2007b) Selection bias between two Medicare capitated benefit programs, *American Journal of Managed Care*, 13(4), 201–207.

Leutz, W. and Greenlick, M. (1995) Reply to Manton *et al.*, *Medical Care*, 33(12), 1228–1231.

Leutz, W. and Greenlick, M. (1998) *The Social HMO Demonstration: Myths and Realities Reconsidered*. Available online via http://socialhmo.brandeis.edu/

Leutz, W. and Ikegami, N. (2004) Coordinating medical care and long-term care: field report from Japan, *International Journal of Integrated Care*. Available online via http://www.ijic.org/newsletter/

Malone, J. *et al.* (2004) *MSHO Care Coordination Study: Final Report.* St. Paul, MN, Minnesota Department of Human Services.

Manton, K. *et al.* (1993) Social/health maintenance organization and fee-for-service outcomes over time, *Health Care Financing Review*, 15(2), 174–202.

Mays, N. (1997) *Total Purchasing: A Profile of National Pilot Projects.* London, Kings Fund.

MSHO (2007) *Minnesota Senior Health Options.* Minnesota Department of Health Services. Available online via http://www.dhs.state.mn.us/main/idcplg?IdcService=GET_DYNAMIC_CONVERSION

Myles, S. *et al.* (1997) *National Evaluation of Total Purchasing Pilot Schemes: Community and Continuing Care for People with Complex Needs.* Report to the UK Department of Health, Total Purchasing National Evaluation Team.

Newcomer, R. (1993) *Service Use and Expenditures in the Social/Health Maintenance Organization Demonstration.* Report to HCFA.

Newcomer, R. *et al.* (1995) Case mix controlled service use and expenditures in the social/health maintenance organization demonstration, *Journal of Gerontology – Medical Sciences*, 50A(1), M35–M44.

Newcomer, R. *et al.* (1996) Health plan satisfaction and risk of disenrollment among Social/HMO and fee-for-service recipients members of the social health maintenance organization, *Inquiry*, 33(2), 144–154.

Rosenbaum, S. (2000) The Olmstead decision: implications for state health policy, *Health Affairs*, 19(5), 228–232.

Walsh, E. *et al.* (2006) *Design of Evaluation Options of the System Change Grants.* Waltham, MA, RTI International.

WPP (2007) *Wisconsin Partnership Program.* Wisconsin Department of Health and Family Services. Available online via http://dhfs.wisconsin.gov/wipartnership/

4 Key elements in effective partnership working

Henk Nies

This chapter deals with a key element of effective partnerships: systems and processes. In other words, what systems need to be in place and how can they be implemented? However, before addressing the effectiveness of systems and processes, it is necessary to be clear about the definition of the term 'effective' (see also Chapter 11). The answer to this question is a normative one. In this context, it is assumed that the main objective of partnership working is to meet the needs of service users with complex, long-lasting problems: the target group of long-term care. This may be frail older people, older people suffering from a disabling disease (such as dementia), people with ongoing needs from a disabling disease or who have not yet recovered from such a disease (e.g. stroke), people with complex psychiatric symptoms (e.g. schizophrenia) or people with learning disabilities. Similar issues may also arise for other groups (e.g. young people with behavioural and social problems).

What all these groups have in common is that they suffer from a mix of acute and chronic medical problems, as well as functional disabilities. Moreover, their support networks are frequently overburdened (Johri *et al.*, 2003; Saltman *et al.*, 2006) and they often experience difficulties in various aspects of their daily living. Elsewhere we have characterised the group that may benefit most from fully integrated services – or partnership working – as people with complex, multiple 'messy' problems; severe levels of dependency; unstable, unpredictable conditions; a need for a range of services; a need for high-intensity service provision; long-term or terminal needs; and a weak sense of self-direction (Nies, 2006). At the same time, it can be argued that effective partnership working should meet the objectives that are widely used within the European Union (EU) with regard to health care systems; it should provide good quality care, be accessible and be financially sustainable (Commission of the European Communities, 2003; OECD, 2005).

What do we mean by 'quality of life'?

In contemporary thinking, the traditional disease-oriented view of human functioning is often seen as too limited, and a view that emphasises quality of life appears to be more suitable. For this purpose, we follow a World Health Organization (WHO) definition of long-term care as:

> The system of activities undertaken by informal caregivers (family, friends and/or neighbours) and/or professionals (health and social services) to ensure that a person who is not fully capable of self-care can maintain the highest possible quality of life, according to his or her individual preferences, with the greatest possible degree of independence, autonomy, participation, personal fulfilment and human dignity. (WHO, 2000)

This implies that the effectiveness of partnership working should be assessed against the extent to which it delivers quality of life. While there is a large body of literature on this topic, this chapter adopts a framework based on work by Petzoldt (1994, in Houben, 2002) and Schalock and Verdugo-Alonso (2002). The work of these authors formed the basis of the performance indicators that have been developed for long-term care services in the Netherlands (ActiZ et al., 2006; VGN, 2007). The key elements are summarised in Figure 4.1.

The model demonstrates the central role of self-direction: the autonomy of the person to follow his or her preferences to achieve a good physical and mental health condition, optimum social relationships, material well-being, personal fulfilment, social participation and meeting individual goals and aspirations. Given the breadth of this model, the social and physical environment has a key role to play alongside policy and broader society either in helping to achieve such a vision or in acting as a barrier.

Above all, the model implies that effective partnership working should be based on user involvement, with the values and preferences of the individual taken as a key point of departure (see also Chapter 9 on the concept of self-care). As a result, the model includes a series of relevant domains of life and living conditions, such as social relationships, health, education, work, housing and income.

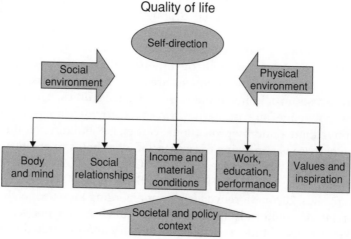

Figure 4.1 Quality of life in long-term care.

As a consequence, partnership working should focus on two different types of relationship:

1. The relationship between self-care, informal care and professional care.
2. The relationship between different aspects of formal service provision within the health care sector (including long-term care, acute care, public health, rehabilitation and mental health) and across sectors (including housing, technology, neighbourhood development, social care, welfare, work, leisure, education and social protection).

Clearly these are ambitious aims, and most developed countries are struggling to deliver these aspirations in full and in practice.

International evidence and theory

Elements of integration

Over the past 10–20 years a growing body of literature has emerged on partnership working and related concepts such as integrated care, disease management, whole systems working, managed care, chronic illness management and chain management (to name but a few key terms). While disease-oriented models primarily provide protocols for health care providers in treating specific diseases, chronic care, disability or gerontological models are often more suited for responding to chronic conditions, co-morbidity and functional impairments within their social and physical context. These latter approaches are therefore more appropriate for groups with diffuse, multiple problems, such as frail older people (Hollander Feldman and Kane, 2003; Leichsenring, 2004a; Lynch et al., 2005).

For long-term care there are very few, well-developed care pathways. Whereas supply chain management models may be appropriate with regards to disease management, other paradigms may be better suited to long-term care: tailoring support to the needs of the individual, dealing with and accepting logistical complexities, ensuring coherent interventions and support, focusing on the quality of the relationship between care recipient and care worker, and reorganising care to connect what is relevant and to apply operational values (Schumacher et al., 2006).

The formal evidence on what elements are effective in partnership working in long-term care rests on a limited number of controlled studies. In contrast, the current body of knowledge relies primarily on insights provided by case studies – often of a descriptive kind – and by professional consensus. Building on these sources of knowledge, there is a growing awareness of what helps to create and sustain effective partnerships working (see, e.g., Audit Commission, 2002; Johri et al., 2003; Leichsenring and Alaszewski, 2004; Nies and Berman, 2004; van Exel et al., 2005; Kodner, 2006; Nies, 2006). Moreover, from our emerging knowledge, these factors seem to be relatively uniformly applicable across different systems (see Figure 4.2).

Ideally, key factors include a single point of entry and integrated needs assessments, leading to integrated care or service plans, with care and services being

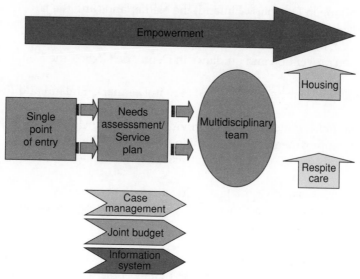

Figure 4.2 Factors contributing to effective partnerships.

delivered by integrated multidisciplinary teams, and supported by case or care management, joint budgets and integrated information systems (Johri *et al.*, 2003; OECD, 2005; Kodner, 2006). Less rigorously evaluated, but still promising, are approaches which include adequate housing, as well as specific combinations of housing, welfare and care, short breaks to support family carers and mechanisms to increase older people's self-direction (e.g. personal budgets; see Chapter 10). Moreover, the combination of the full range of these key elements is likely to be stronger than merely summing up their single effects (Johri *et al.*, 2003). Despite this, more research is needed to establish exactly which groups of service users may benefit most from these arrangements and for which groups such arrangements may not be effective. Furthermore, little is known about the extent to which it is possible for partner agencies to pursue both depth and breadth of organisational relationships at the same time (Glasby, 2005, 2007; see also the Introduction to this book).

Both in Europe and in North America, many of the key elements of partnership working – or as it is usually referred to in the international literature, integrated care – are on the policy agenda and are being implemented. There is wide awareness of the need for coherent and continuous service delivery and, hence, for integrating services; however, the exact wording and the policy context differs from country to country. An overview by Leichsenring (2004b) has highlighted (without striving towards completeness and methodological perfection) a number of elements of integration in a number of EU member states:

- Case and care management in Denmark, Finland, the Netherlands and the UK.
- Multi-professional needs assessment and joint planning in Denmark, Finland, France, Ireland, the Netherlands and the UK.

- Joint working in Denmark, Finland, the Netherlands and the UK.
- Consumer-directed services (personal budgets, long-term care insurance) in Austria, Germany, Finland and the Netherlands.
- Admission prevention and guidance in Denmark, Greece, the Netherlands and the UK.
- Integration of housing, welfare and care in Denmark, Finland and the Netherlands.
- Integration of family carers into provider systems (including targeted respite schemes, employment, etc.) in Germany, France and Finland.
- Independent advice, support and care coordination in Germany and the Netherlands.
- Case conferences to coordinate care in Denmark and the UK.
- Integrated quality management and assurance systems in Germany, France, Finland, Ireland and the UK.

While many EU member states claim to be reforming their systems to ensure continuity and coherence of care to support older people to stay in the community for as long as possible, many current policies are only partially implemented at the national level. Apart from policies to ensure the financial sustainability of welfare systems (and long-term care in particular), measures are being taken to improve system performance. A crucial issue here is the importance of support for informal carers, as informal care covers an estimated 80–90% of all care that is provided to older people. Moreover, front-line services are also being re-designed in a number of countries, particularly with regards to the relationships between health and social care and between home and community care. Broader developments also include the creation of purpose-built approaches, such as care-friendly districts in the Netherlands and open care centres in Greece (OECD, 2005; Saltman et al., 2006). At the same time, many countries have developed cash payment programmes in lieu of or in conjunction with services in kind in order to strengthen consumer direction and choice (Lundsgaard, 2005; Timonen et al., 2006; see also Chapter 10). However, although policy systems vary with respect to responsibilities and funding mechanisms, the relationship between the system and front-line service delivery is often weak. All systems are facing basically the same problems, particularly when related sectors such as housing and income are included (van Raak et al., 2003; Leichsenring and Alaszewski, 2004; Nies and Berman, 2004; Billings and Leichsenring, 2005). The underlying question is whether health and social care systems as such are a barrier to integration, or whether governing and managing complex systems or organisations always imply fragmentation (Nies, 2007; see also Chapter 3).

Organisational structures

These elements of integration or partnership working are implemented in a wide variety of organisational or – more accurately – inter-organisational structures. Particularly crucial is the way in which appropriate interconnections are ensured: between the service user, informal carer and professional; between various aspects of the health care system (such as long-term care, acute care, public health, rehabilitation and mental health); and across all relevant sectors (e.g. housing, technology, neighbourhood development, social care, welfare, leisure, education and social protection). Leutz's (1999) distinction between three types of integration – 'linkage', 'coordination' and 'full integration' – are well known (see Chapter 3), and these have similarities to Glasby's (2007) depth and breadth matrix (see the Introduction to this book). However, Pieper (2004) also helpfully distinguishes between 'integrated organisations' and 'integrated networks'. By bringing together functions into a single hierarchy, integrated organisations are formal, free-standing entities with scope to integrate services directly within their control. However, integrated networks depend more on developing integrated approaches between essentially independent partners. While this may enable individual organisations to meet their own interests (and may be less disruptive than full integration), such relationships can also reveal differences in terms of values, interests and goals. This in turn can result in costs, risks and potential conflict that call for negotiation, compromise and trust. Building on this analysis, Pieper (2005) strongly argues that integration – or partnership working – typically involves a continuous process of balancing: of power and influence; of quality versus costs; of benefits, costs and risks; and of self-interest versus social justice.

Within the organisation of integrated service delivery, six interfaces have to be resolved (Pieper, 2005):

1. The integration of professional care and service provision with everyday life and with the interests and choices of service users.
2. Specific tasks have to be assigned to relevant managers and professionals.
3. Tasks have to be coordinated, and this coordination has to be assigned and agreed upon as well.
4. Services have to be coordinated, which usually implies mediating inter-organisational relationships (case management may be such a coordinating mechanism).
5. The interests of organisations have to be balanced which requires governance codes, procedures and structures, often involving a third party to provide a degree of stability (see, e.g., Kaats *et al.*, 2005).
6. Integration of the 'higher' levels of partnership organisation in the policy system through adequate legal and financial arrangements and contracts. This requires a system of well-designed levers and incentives.

All this analysis implies that processes need to be integrated at various levels: individual, organisational and structural/system level (Pieper, 2005; see also the Introduction to this book). Moreover, the intensity and spectrum of connections differ across these levels and according to the complexity of the needs of the user groups concerned. Leutz (1999) has tentatively depicted some of these relationships (see Table 4.1, based on Leutz, 1999, and Nies, 2004).

However, little is known about which organisational structures are most appropriate for which types of service users. In general, it is safe to suggest that the structure should enable support with regards to all domains of life in which

Table 4.1 Levels of integration.

Client's needs	Linkage	Coordination	Full integration
Severity	Mild to moderate	Moderate to severe	Moderate to severe
Stability	Stable	Stable	Unstable
Duration	Short- to long-term	Short- to long-term	Long-term to terminal
Urgency	Routine or non-urgent	Mostly routine	Frequent, urgent
Scope of services	Narrow to moderate	Moderate to broad	Broad
Self-direction	Self-directed or strong informal	Varied levels of self-direction	Weak self-direction or informal

Adapted from Leutz (1999).

people are dependent on external support or with which therapeutic interventions are required. The organisation of services should thus follow and anticipate the needs of the service user.

For partnership working, the inter-organisational dimension is particularly relevant. Links, coordinating mechanisms or integrated structures are required to follow and anticipate the needs of the service user. At group level, the concept of care pathways defines strategies of integration among the various services and practitioners involved. Care pathways are primarily developed in the acute health care sector. However, they may be helpful in long-term care as well in order to optimise continuity of care, to specify responsibilities and resources and to involve the person and his or her family in the process of care and service delivery (see, e.g., Murray *et al.*, 2005). A care pathway can be conceived as a sequence of multiple decisions to be made based on appropriate and – as far as possible – evidence-based interventions for a specific target group, supported by guidelines and monitored by scores on relevant indicators (Vecchiato, 2004).

Care pathways follow a (cyclic) process of:

- awareness raising among service users and their social network;
- exploration of the problem: needs assessment, diagnostics, etc.;
- planning the intervention (care or support): assessing eligibility and allocating resources, based on an individualised care/support plan and, at group level, on a care pathway;
- delivery of care and services: in partnership, usually by a multidisciplinary and multi-organisational team;
- evaluation and adjustment.

While these steps – or elements – are designed to meet the needs of the service user, they can also be conceived (from an organisational perspective) as links in a chain, each having a strategic value for the various participating organisations. de Bruijn and ten Heuvelhof (1999) present a number of such links:

- *Selecting link*-it determines what happens in the next stages. In the care sector this is often the professional or agency that is responsible for assessment and/or diagnostics (e.g. general practitioners, social workers, single points of entry, diagnostic centres (for instance, memory clinics), assessment committees and gatekeepers of service delivery in general).

- *Allocating link*-it also determines what happens in the next stages, but has a say or strong influence on resource allocation. This is often synonymous with the selecting link, but not always. It can be a planning or coordinating agency but also a health care insurer who decides on budgets.
- *Weakest link*-it provides insufficient quality and information or insufficient resources; inputs and outputs may stagnate, affecting the whole chain.
- *Narrow link*-only a few actors are crucial here (for instance, because of the specificity of their profession, specific consultants); these links are vulnerable because they depend on a limited number of people. Individual factors strongly influence the quality of the narrow link.
- *Broad link*-many actors are relevant here (for instance, because of the more general focus of their profession – e.g. general practitioners or social workers). These links can be difficult to manage because of the number of key people involved and because of the potential breadth of their focus.

In particular, these distinctions help to explore and understand the strategic behaviour of managers in inter-agency settings. Thus, the selecting and allocating links are crucial to influence the whole local or regional system, the weakest link should be eliminated or compensated, the narrow link should be well organised and used appropriately, and the broad link should be engaged through key opinion leaders.

The difficult and arduous thing about partnership working is the need to organise these dynamics and key elements in a way that provides coherence and continuity to service users and informal carers. As suggested earlier, current health and social care systems are highly fragmented in terms of funding, legislation, organisation, culture and working practices. Case or care management is often seen as a useful mechanism to overcome these barriers. However, more joined-up funding and information systems across systems are also required. While specific details may differ from country to country (see Esping-Anderson, 1990, on different types of welfare regime), the need for these underlying mechanisms seems relatively universal across all Western welfare states. Moreover, cross-cutting studies of the process of integration (see, e.g., Mur-Veeman *et al.*, 2000; Eijkelberg, 2007) have concluded that an interplay of power, culture and leadership determines to a large extent how partnerships at regional level develop.

Implications and conclusions

In summary, partnership working will never be an easy task, as many services' core business is the provision of monodisciplinary tasks. However, the ageing of the population calls for integrative mechanisms, since many service users suffer from multiple problems and since single interventions are frequently insufficient. As a result, both horizontal and vertical models of management are required, together with matrix structures (with all their complexities) that enable the provision of both single and multiple interventions. To cite Walter Leutz (1999; see also Chapter 3):

> You can integrate all of the services for some of the people, or some of the services for all of the people, but you can't integrate all of the services for all of the people.

Summary

- For people with complex, multiple and ongoing needs, a traditional disease-oriented approach to service delivery is insufficient. Instead, a range of services will be required, depending on the needs of the individual.
- Effective partnership working should seek to boost quality of life, focusing on key service user outcomes across the various domains of life.
- In developing partnerships, it is important not to overlook the contribution of family (or informal) carers.
- Thus, partnerships need to achieve integration between service users, informal carers and professionals; between all relevant sectors of the health care system; and between different sectors (including housing, technology, neighbourhood development, social care, welfare, work, education and social protection).
- Key elements include a single point of entry, integrated needs assessments, integrated care or service plans and services delivered via integrated, multidisciplinary teams, often supported by case or care management, joint budgets and integrated information systems.
- Effective partnership has to take place at three different levels: that of the individual, the organisation and the policy system and structures by which services are governed. Within these levels, a series of different interfaces between policy, practice and the individual need to be considered.
- At group level, care pathways can specify the integration of the various services and practitioners, optimising continuity of care, specifying responsibilities and resources, and involving the person and his or her family in the process of care and service delivery.
- Developing partnership structures requires input from multiple actors. Within this an interplay of power, culture and leadership is a key determinant.
- Key mechanisms to support partnership working seem to be relatively universal across different systems.

Further reading and useful websites

For literature on the management of integrated care, see:
Nies, H. and Berman, P. (eds) (2004) *Integrating Services for Older People: A Resource Book from European Experience*. Dublin, European Health Management Association.

For an overview of EU and OECD long-term care policies, see:

Lundsgaard, J. (2005) *Consumer Direction and Choice in Long-Term Care for Older Persons, Including Payments for Informal Care: How Can It Help Improve Care Outcomes, Employment and Fiscal Sustainability?* Paris, OECD.

OECD (2005) *Long-Term Care for Older People.* Paris, OECD.

For a European overview and practice examples in EU members states (as well as a conceptual analysis), see:

Alaszewski, A., Billings, J. and Coxon, K. (2004) Integrated health and social care for older persons: theoretical and conceptual issues, in K. Leichsenring and A. Alaszewski (eds) *Providing Integrated Health and Social Care for Older Persons: A European Overview of Issues at Stake.* Abingdon, Ashgate.

Billings, J. and Leichsenring, K. (eds) (2005) *Integrating Health and Social Care Services for Older Persons: Evidence from Nine European Countries.* Abingdon, Ashgate.

van Raak, A. *et al.* (eds) (2003) *Integrated Care in Europe: Description and Comparison of Integrated Care in Six EU Countries.* Maarssen, Elsevier Gezondheidszorg.

For an overview of ageing in Europe and its consequences, see:

European Commission (2007) *Europe's Demographic Future: Facts and Figures.* Brussels, SEC(2007) 638.

European Commission (2008) Long-term care in the European Union. Brussels: DG Employment, Social Affairs and Equal Opportunities.

Relevant websites include:

The *International Journal of Integrated Care* is a free online journal with articles on theory, research, policy and projects. The journal also organises annual conferences: http://www.ijic.org

CARMEN (the Care and Management of Services for Older People in Europe Network, commissioned by the European Commission) contains a number of key resources, including the web book: Nies, H. and Berman, P. (eds) (2004) *Integrating Services for Older People: A Resource Book from European Experience.* Dublin, European Health Management Association: http://www.ehma.org/carmen/index.html

PROCARE (Providing Health and Social Care for Older Persons: issues, problems and solutions), commissioned by the European Commission, has a website with key reports and presentations from this European project: http://www.euro.centre.org/procare/

EUROFAMCARE provides rich materials on informal care or family care in 23 European countries and extensive research data on 6 of these countries: http://www.uke.uni-hamburg.de/extern/eurofamcare/

Eurocarers is a European organisation working for carers. The website contains a series of guiding principles to support informal care in the community: http://www.eurocarers.org/

References

ActiZ *et al.* (2006) *Kwaliteitskader Verantwoorde Zorg* (Quality framework to ensure responsible care; in Dutch). Utrecht, Stuurgroep Verantwoorde Zorg. Available online via http://www.zorgvoorbeter.nl/docs/Kwaliteitskader_Verantwoorde_Zorg_VVT_2007.pdf

Audit Commission (2002) *Integrated Services for Older People: Building a Whole System Approach in England*. London, Audit Commission.

Billings, J. and Leichsenring, K. (eds) (2005) *Integrating Health and Social Care Services for Older Persons: Evidence from Nine European Countries*. Abingdon, Ashgate.

Commission of the European Communities (2003) *Health Care and Care for the Elderly: Supporting National Strategies for Ensuring a High Level of Social Protection*. Communication from the Commission to the Council, the European Parliament, the European Economic and Social Committee and the Committee of the Region.

de Bruijn, J.A. and ten Heuvelhof, E.F. (1999) *Management in Netwerken*, 2nd edn (Management in Networks; in Dutch). Utrecht, Lemma.

Eijkelberg, I. (2007) *Key Factors of Change Processes in Shared Care: Viewpoints of Managers, Care Providers and Patients*. PhD thesis, University of Maastricht.

Esping-Anderson, G. (1990) *The Three Worlds of Welfare Capitalism*. Cambridge, Polity Press.

Glasby, J. (2005) The integration dilemma: how deep and how broad to go? *Journal of Integrated Care*, 13(5), 27–30.

Glasby, J. (2007) *Understanding Health and Social Care*. Bristol, Policy Press.

Hollander Feldman, P. and Kane, R. (2003) Strengthening research to improve the practice and management of long-term care, *The Milbank Quarterly*, 81(2), 179–220.

Houben, P.P.J. (2002) *Levensloopbeleid: Interactief Levensloopbeleid Ontwerpen in de Tweede Levenshelft*. (Life-cycle oriented policies: interactive life-cycle oriented policy developments in the second half of life) Maarssen, Elsevier.

Johri, M., Béland, F. and Bergman, H. (2003) International experiments in integrated care for the elderly: a synthesis of the evidence, *International Journal of Geriatric Psychiatry*, 18, 222–235.

Kaats, E., van Klaveren, P. and Opheij, W. (2005) *Organiseren Tussen Organisaties* (Organising between organisations; in Dutch). Schiedam, Scriptum.

Kodner, D.L. (2006) Whole-system approaches to health and social care partnerships for the frail elderly: an exploration of North American models and lessons, *Health and Social Care in the Community*, 14(5), 384–390.

Leichsenring, K. (2004a) Developing integrated health and social care services for older persons in Europe, *International Journal of Integrated Care*, 4. Available online via http://www.ijic.org

Leichsenring, K. (2004b) Providing integrated health and social care: a European overview, in K. Leichsenring and A. Alaszewski (eds) *Providing Integrated Health and Social Care for Older Persons: A European Overview of Issues at Stake*. Abingdon, Ashgate.

Leichsenring, K. and Alaszewski, A. (Eds) (2004) *Providing Integrated Health and Social Care for Older Persons: A European Overview of Issues at Stake*. Ashgate, Aldershot.

Leutz, W. (1999) Five laws for integrating medical and social services: lessons from the US and the UK, *Milbank Quarterly*, 77(1), 77–110.

Lundsgaard, J. (2005) *Consumer Direction and Choice in Long-Term Care for Older Persons, Including Payments for Informal Care: How Can It Help Improve Care Outcomes, Employment and Fiscal Sustainability?* Paris, OECD.

Lynch, M., Estes, C.L. and Hernandez, M. (2005) Chronic care initiatives for the elderly: can they bridge the gerontology–medicine gap? *Journal of Applied Gerontology*, 24(2), 108–124.

Mur-Veeman, I.M., Eijkelberg, I. and Spreeuwenberg, C. (2000) How to manage the implementation of shared care: a discussion of the role of power, culture and structure in the development of shared care arrangements, *Journal of Management in Medicine*, 15(2), 142–155.

Murray, S.A. *et al.* (2005) Illness trajectories and palliative care, *British Medical Journal*, 330, 1007–1011.

Nies, H. (2004) Integrated care: concepts and background, in H. Nies and P. Berman (eds) *Integrating Services for Older People: A Resource Book from European Experience*. Dublin, European Health Management Association.

Nies, H. (2006) Managing effective partnerships in older people's services, *Health and Social Care in the Community*, 14(5), 391–399.

Nies, H. (2007) *Integrated Care for Older People: Is It Happening in Practice?* Paper presented at the 10th European Health Forum, Gastein.

Nies, H. and Berman, P. (eds) (2004) *Integrating Services for Older People: A Resource Book from European Experience*. Dublin, European Health Management Association.

OECD (2005) *Long-Term Care for Older People*. Paris, OECD.

Petzold, H. (1994) Kreatieve Persönlichkeitsdiagnostik durch 'mediengestützte Techniken' in der Integrativen Therapie und Beratung', *Integratieve Therapie*, 4, 340–391.

Pieper, R. (2004) Integrated organisational structures, in H. Nies and P. Berman (eds) *Integrating Services for Older People: A Resource Book from European Experience*. Dublin, European Health Management Association.

Pieper, R. (2005) Integrated care: concepts and theoretical notions, in M. Vaarama and R. Pieper (eds) *Managing Integrated Care for Older Persons*. Helsinki/Dublin, Stakes/EHMA.

Saltman, R.B., Dubois, H.F.W. and Mukesh, C. (2006) The impact of aging on long-term care in Europe and some potential policy responses, *International Journal of Health Services*, 36(4), 719–746.

Schalock, R.L. and Verdugo-Alonso, M.A. (2002) *Handbook on Quality of Life for Human Services Practitioners*. Washington, American Association for Mental Retardation.

Schumacher, J., Konijn, T. and Nies, H. (2006) *Ketens in de Langdurige Zorg* (Chains in long-term care; in Dutch). Utrecht, Lemma.

Timonen, V., Convery, J. and Cahill, S. (2006) Care revolutions in the making? A comparison of cash-for-care programmes in four European countries, *Ageing and Society*, 26, 455–474.

van Exel, N.J.A. *et al.* (2005) Cost effectiveness of integrated stroke services: a prospective study in 411 Dutch patients, *QJM*, 98, 415–425.

van Raak, A. *et al.* (eds) (2003) *Integrated Care in Europe: Description and Comparison of Integrated Care in Six EU Countries*. Maarssen, Elsevier Gezondheidszorg.

Vecchiato, T. (2004) Care pathways, in H. Nies and P. Berman (eds) *Integrating Services for Older People: A Resource Book from European Experience*. Dublin, European Health Management Association.

VGN (2007) *Kwaliteitskader Gehandicaptenzorg* (Visiedocument) (Framework for quality care in the field of services for people with disabilities; in Dutch). Utrecht, Vereniging Gehandicaptenzorg Nederland. Available online via http://62.25.2.16/274616/Visiedocument_kwaliteitskad1.pdf

World Health Organization (WHO) (2000) *Towards an International Consensus on Policy for Long-term Care for the Ageing*. World Health Organisation and Milbank Memorial Fund.

5 Integrated service models: an exploration of North American models and lessons[1]

Dennis Kodner

Irrespective of cross-national differences in long-term care, many developed countries confront broadly similar challenges, including fragmented services, disjointed care, less than optimal quality, system inefficiencies and difficult-to-control costs (Kodner, 2004). Against this backdrop, integrated or whole system strategies are becoming increasingly important to address these shortcomings through the seamless provision of health and social care. This chapter summarises the structure, features and outcomes of key models of service integration in North America, identifying a somewhat positive pattern of results in terms of service access, utilisation, costs, care provision, quality, health status and client/carer satisfaction. It concludes with the identification of common characteristics which are thought to be associated with the successful impact of these integration initiatives, as well as a call for further research to understand the relationships, if any, between whole system models, services and outcomes.

While the move towards greater partnership working is apparent in services for a range of different user groups, this chapter focuses on the example of services for the frail elderly. At the present moment in time, countries around the world are experiencing the broad societal consequences of population ageing, including chronic illness and disability (Kodner, 2003). It is within this context that long-term care for disabled people, particularly the elderly, has become a significant public concern (Jacobzone, 1999). This concern is heightened by growing demands for long-term care services and ever-present budget constraints (OECD, 2005). Long-term care is part health care and part social service. It encompasses a broad array of services delivered in home, community or institutional settings by paid professionals and paraprofessionals – as well as unpaid family carers and other 'informal' helpers – to frail and disabled individuals with complex, multifaceted problems who need assistance with activities of daily living on a prolonged basis. This assistance includes personal care, household chores and life management activities,

---

[1]This chapter is an updated version of a journal article by the same author which first appeared in *Health and Social Care in the Community* (2006), 14(5), 384–390.

often entailing interaction with various parts of the medical, mental health, housing and income maintenance systems (Feder *et al.*, 2000; WHO and Milbank Memorial Fund, 2000).

Despite cross-national differences in policy, funding, infrastructure and provision, many developed countries are actively exploring whole system approaches to long-term care (Kodner, 2002). At the core of these efforts is 'integrated care', defined by Kodner and Spreeuwenberg (2002) as a 'discrete set of techniques and organisational models designed to create connectivity, alignment, and collaboration within and between the cure and care sectors at the funding, administrative and/or provider levels'. As a result of its growing policy prominence, there is an expanding body of literature on various whole system models of long-term care partnership working, particularly prototypes that are nested in single structures designed to more or less tie together health and social care 'under one roof' (see, e.g., Kodner and Kay Kyriacou, 2000; Kodner, 2002, 2004; Johri *et al.*, 2003). Yet, there is also an increasing sense, most frequently articulated in the UK, that more is known about how well these integrated approaches effect the partnership process (i.e. how agencies work together) than the impact they have on the services and outcomes resulting for clients and carers (Dowling *et al.*, 2004; see also Chapter 11).

Varied programmes and demonstrations in integrated care for the elderly are found in a number of countries (see, e.g., Kodner, 2002; Glasby and Peck, 2003; Johri *et al.*, 2003). However, North America is an especially fertile proving ground for whole system approaches. Well-known models include PACE (Program of All-Inclusive Care for the Elderly) and Social HMOs (Health Maintenance Organisations) in the US, and SIPA (in French, *Système de soins Intégrés pour Personnes Âgées*), PRISMA (Programme of Research to Integrate Services for the Maintenance of Autonomy) and CHOICE (Comprehensive Home Option of Integrated Care for the Elderly) in Canada. The experiences of the successful PACE, SIPA and PRISMA models, in particular, can shed important light on 'what works and under what circumstances' in whole system approaches to integrated care for the frail elderly.

Descriptions and results of three successful models

The following section summarises the structure, major features and outcomes of the PACE, SIPA and PRISMA programmes, including their impact on service utilisation, costs, care provision and health outcomes. Some of these examples, themes and issues are also picked up in contributions by Walter Leutz (Chapter 3) and Helen Dickinson (Chapter 11), as well as by other contributors in subsequent chapters.

PACE (US)

PACE is a fully integrated system that provides acute and long-term care services which are coordinated by, and largely organised around, an adult day health centre. The model grew out of On Lok, an innovative senior centre, which, starting in 1971, began to gradually adapt the British day-hospital approach to the care of the frail elderly in San Francisco's Chinatown (Eng et al., 1997). The adult day health centre setting, in addition to offering social and respite services, functions largely as a geriatric outpatient clinic in which primary medical care, ongoing clinical oversight and care management play major roles. The programme is designed to maintain frail older people in the community for as long as possible, as well as to avoid or postpone institutionalisation through effective, community-based geriatric care (Bodenheimer, 1999). Enrolment, which is voluntary, is targeted to community-dwelling elderly people aged 55 and over who are eligible for nursing home admission and covered by both Medicare (the federal health insurance programme for the elderly and people with disabilities) and Medicaid (the joint federal–state, means-tested health care programme for low-income and medically indigent individuals). The involvement of informal carers is emphasised and supportive housing, though not a formal benefit, is frequently used as an important adjunct to the care package (Kodner and Kay Kyriacou, 2000). PACE operated as a federal demonstration programme between 1987 and 1997, and is currently a permanent provider under Medicare and a state option under Medicaid. As of January 2005, there were 36 fully operational programmes in 18 states caring for 10 523 enrolees (National PACE Association, 2005a). According to the National PACE Association, the typical participant is very similar to the average American nursing home resident: she is 80 years old, has 9.7 medical conditions and is limited in approximately three activities of daily living; 49% have been diagnosed with dementia (National PACE Association, 2005b).

The PACE model achieves integration on several levels:

1. Financing through the pooling of Medicare and Medicaid revenues along with total control over all programme expenditures and the authority to use these prepaid, capitated funds flexibly.
2. Service delivery largely provided by the staff of the adult day health centre with outside contracts for specialty medical services, acute hospitalisation and nursing home care.
3. Case management by a multidisciplinary team responsible for comprehensive assessment, service provision and arrangement, care coordination and clinical monitoring.
4. A focus on prevention, rehabilitation and other clinical and system efficiencies driven by consolidated service delivery and risk-based capitation (Ansak, 1990).

The US Health Care Financing Administration (now known as the Centers for Medicare and Medicaid) commissioned both qualitative (Kane et al., 1992) and a quantitative evaluations conducted by a team of researchers at Abt Associates (1993–1998). The latter employed non-randomised, quasi-experimental designs. Both Kane et al. (1992) and Zimmerman et al. (1998) found the PACE model to be very effective as an integrating mechanism. The intense geriatric focus, use of the adult day health centre as the combined setting for primary medical care, health, social and supportive services, and the team aspects of the programme were singled out as being most responsible for the programme's highly personalised care and effective clinical coordination and continuity. Enrolment in PACE was also associated with a large decrease in hospital use (both admissions and days), reduced institutionalisation (both admissions and days) and substantial increases in the utilisation of outpatient medical care and therapies, as well as home- and community-based services (Chatterji *et al.*, 1998). There was also a positive impact on Medicare costs vis-à-vis the non-enrolee comparison group (White, 1998). In addition, Chatterji *et al.* (1998) found favourable measures in terms of client health status and overall satisfaction with care arrangements. However, results in terms of physical functioning were inconsistent, and no statistically significant differences in quality of life were observed between comparison groups.

The above results suggest that PACE is successful in managing frail elderly patients in the community and in offsetting more expensive inpatient services (Eng *et al.*, 1997; Chatterji *et al.*, 1998). However, Kodner and Kay Kyriacou (2000) point to several unique features which impose a self-limiting effect on the growth of the programme. Firstly, without the assistance of the federal and state governments, substantial capital and start-up costs in millions of dollars are difficult to fund privately. Secondly, some elderly applicants do not end up joining the programme because they are not comfortable with the adult day health care setting or with the fact that they must give up their personal physician for on-site primary care. Thirdly, the small size of the centre sites (averaging 300 enrolees) presents an economy of scale issue in terms of widespread national replication.

SIPA (Canada)

Like the American PACE programme, the Quebec-based SIPA demonstration is another example of a fully integrated model of care. The originators of this model at the McGill University/Université de Montréal Research Group on Integrated Services for the Frail Elderly describe SIPA as a community-based, primary care-led, case-managed health system for the frail elderly (Bergman *et al.*, 1997). The project was carried out at two Montréal CLSCs (in French, *Centres de Locaux de Services Communitaires*) over a 22-month period between June 1999 and March 2001. The CLSC is a local, publicly run community clinic which is also responsible for home care in the province of Quebec (Trahan and Caris, 2002). The two CLSC-based SIPA teams, each operating with their own management, budget and staff, were responsible for the integrated provision of community health and social services and the coordination of hospital and nursing home care for 160 patients per site (Bergman *et al.*, 2003). Enrolment in the programme was limited to community-dwelling elderly people aged 64 and over residing in the CLSC demonstration areas with moderate disability and the willingness of carer(s) to participate. Most health care and community services were provided directly by the CLSC, with hospitals, nursing homes and other contract providers delivering more specialised services (Hollander *et al.*, 2002).

In addition to the basic demonstration design outlined earlier, several other major features are associated with the model (Bergman *et al.*, 1997; Johri *et al.*, 2003):

1. A multidisciplinary team, consisting of the participant's personal physician, nurses or social workers (acting as case managers), therapists, home care workers and sometimes nutritionists and pharmacists, assumes total clinical responsibility in all settings.
2. A battery of evidence-based geriatric techniques, including multidisciplinary clinical protocols, intensive home care, 24-hour on-call availability and rapid team mobilisation, are used to minimise functional decline, reduce inappropriate institutionalisation and maintain community living for as long as possible.
3. Payment based on prepaid capitation is designed to ensure responsibility for the full range of health and social services covered by the programme. (NB: Prepaid financing was never implemented as part of the demonstration, although SIPA retained the flexible use of funds for all community-based medical and social care and staff were made aware of relative costs, thus attempting to simulate its effects.)

The SIPA demonstration is the only known randomised control trial (RCT) of a North American integrated model of care for the elderly. The results reported by Béland *et al.* (2006) show that the programme was highly effective in increasing access to community-based health and social services and reducing the acute hospitalisations (by 50%) of alternate level of care patients (i.e. 'bed blockers' who are chronically ill and disabled). While positive patterns were discerned in overall hospital and nursing home use, no significant differences in emergency department, hospital or nursing home stays or costs were found. Moreover, there were no differences in health outcomes or total costs between experimental and control groups. Finally, an increase in carer satisfaction was observed in SIPA without an attendant rise in burden or out-of-pocket costs.

Despite these positive findings, it was decided that SIPA would not become a permanent programme because of the lack of policy consensus. However, the Quebec government is considering the incorporation of certain elements of the model into the province's existing health and social service system (Hollander *et al.*, 2002).

PRISMA (Canada)

Unlike PACE and SIPA, PRISMA is a coordinated model of integrated care. The programme was first pilot tested in the Bois-Francs region of Quebec, and is currently being expanded to the province's Eastern Townships. The goal is to integrate service delivery to ensure clients' functional autonomy. Admission is geared to people who are aged 65 and over who present moderate-to-severe disabilities, show good potential for staying at home, need two or more health care or social services, and live in the service area (Hébert *et al.*, 2005).

The PRISMA model is composed of six main integrating elements (Hébert *et al.*, 2003):

1. Inter- and intra-organisational coordination provided by a joint governing board on the governance level and a service coordination committee on the managerial level.
2. A single point of entry mechanism to access all covered health care and social services in the service area.
3. Clinical management and service coordination through a team of case managers who work with the client's family physician and other providers.
4. A common assessment instrument, clinical chart and care plan.
5. Budgeting of services.
6. An integrated information system, including computerised tools, to automate clinical records, facilitate team work and continuity of care, track participants, and collect clinical and management data.

A quasi-experimental study was undertaken between 1997 and 2003 to evaluate the PRISMA model in the Bois-Francs region. Measurements were taken at 12 months pre-implementation (T1) and every 12 months post-implementation (T2 and T3) (Tourigny *et al.*, 2004). Overall, a declining trend in institutionalisation was observed as well as a lower client preference to be institutionalised. Another important impact was found in terms of functional autonomy, with more frail clients in the study group being maintained at their assessed levels at T1 and T2; however, the effect disappeared at T3. The intervention failed to alter the use of services. Finally, the pilot had a positive effect on carer burden, but not on mortality (survival).

What can we learn about effective whole systems for the frail elderly?

Leutz (2005) maintains that all integration is local (see also Chapter 3). That is, the best of integrated care for the elderly is designed to find specific solutions to local problems. Moreover, success depends, in large part, on local leadership and part-nership working, rather than top-down structural solutions and directives (Hudson *et al.*, 2002). Nonetheless, each programme operates within a national health care and social service context, thus exerting a potentially powerful influence on how models work, both positively and negatively (Johri *et al.*, 2003). Further complicating across-the-board generalisability about programme effectiveness is the ubiquitous heterogeneity in evaluation methodology, including the wide variation in measures used, even for similar indicators and outcomes. This is clearly underscored by the major differences found between the three programmes reviewed in this chapter (see also Chapter 11 for further discussion).

Despite these confounding circumstances, important conclusions can still be drawn about the effectiveness of these North American models, as well as the common characteristics thought to be associated with their success. Table 5.1 presents a summary of the main features of the PACE, SIPA and PRISMA programmes, as well as the principal evaluation findings. The evidence generally points to a promising pattern of outcomes in terms of access, clinical coordination and continuity, functional decline, service utilisation, institutionalisation, quality of life, carer burden and client satisfaction. Although these findings, particularly for PACE and PRISMA, must be viewed somewhat cautiously, it suggests nonetheless that whole system approaches to health and social care partnership based largely on efforts to produce seamless care through forms of structural integration appear to make a difference not only in services, but also in terms of outcomes for users and carers.

Four key elements seem to account for the successful impact of these service initiatives:

1. Umbrella organisational structures guide integration at the strategic, managerial and service delivery levels, encourage and support effective joint working, ensure efficient operations and maintain overall accountability for service, quality and cost outcomes.
2. Case-managed, multidisciplinary team care allows for the effective evaluation and planning of client needs, provides a single contact or entry point into the health care and social service systems, packages and coordinates services, and triages or allocates clinical responsibility.
3. Organised provider networks joined together by standardised referral procedures, service agreements, joint training, shared information systems and even common ownership of resources enhance access to services, provide seamless care and maintain quality.
4. Financial incentives promote prevention, rehabilitation and the downward substitution of services, as well as enable service integration and efficiency.

Effectively integrating long-term health and social care for the frail elderly is an enormously complex and difficult challenge (Leutz, 2005). In addition to combining and successfully implementing the right set of solutions in a meaningful design, numerous bureaucratic, interprofessional and cultural hurdles must be overcome before integrated care bears fruit (and these are explored in other chapters in this book). The PACE programme in the US and the SIPA and PRISMA demonstrations in Canada provide meaningful clues about how and why successful whole system models work, particularly for carers and users. While these initiatives may contain a number of important lessons for other countries, much more work needs to be done to exploit the potentially powerful benefits of integrated care models. This demands greater understanding of the relationships between structures, partnership working, services and results, as well as the need to design organisational, managerial, clinical and other levers that can lead to better services and outcomes for the elderly (Glasby and Littlechild, 2004). In future efforts to measure

Table 5.1   Descriptions and major outcomes of North American programmes and demonstrations.

	PACE (US)	SIPA (Canada)	PRISMA (Canada)
General description	Adult day health centre-based comprehensive health and long-term care programme with risk-based capitation financing for elderly nursing-home-certifiable population	Community-based, primary care-led, case-managed health system for the frail elderly operating out of local community service centres; inspired by PACE	Community-based, case-managed, single point of entry service network
Model type	Fully integrated	Fully integrated	Coordinated
Project objectives	Maintain frail elderly persons in community for as long as possible by avoiding or postponing institutionalisation	Maintain and promote autonomy of frail elderly people, and promote optimal utilisation of community-based services as substitute for hospital and nursing home care	Integrate service delivery to ensure functional autonomy
Target population	1. Community-dwelling elderly residing in service area 2. Aged 55 and over 3. Certification of eligibility for nursing home admission	1. Community-dwelling elderly residing in demonstration area 2. Aged 64 and over 3. Moderate disability 4. Willingness of carer(s) to participate	1. Community-dwelling elderly residing in demonstration area 2. Aged 65 and over 3. Moderate-to-severe impairment 4. Need two or more health care or social services 5. Show good potential for staying at home
Dates	The On Lok model, which is the foundation for PACE, started in 1971. Operated as a federal demonstration between 1987 and 1997. Continues as permanent programme	1999–2001; in two stages	Bois-Franc intervention (1997–1998 to 1998–1999)
Services covered	Comprehensive primary, acute and long-term care; enriched home- and community-based services; on contract basis	Comprehensive long-term care; acute medical and social services, including some respite housing; largely on contract basis	Existing acute, long-term care, rehabilitative and supportive services in region

(Continued)

Table 5.1 *Continued*

	PACE (US)	SIPA (Canada)	PRISMA (Canada)
Service management	Multidisciplinary team, including primary care physicians	Multidisciplinary team working with primary care physicians and others	Case managers working closely with family physicians and others
Size	36 operational sites in 18 states with 10 523 enrolees	1254 persons in two sites; half received SIPA intervention	272 persons (PRISMA cohort); 210 persons (control cohort)
Referral methods	Community outreach; voluntary enrolment	Existing home care clients; referrals from hospitals and physicians, government agencies; outreach activities	Outreach; single point of entry
Payer(s)	Capitated payments from Medicare and Medicaid programmes; some private out-of-pocket premiums	Government	Government
Evaluation methodology	Quasi-experimental, non-randomised design	Randomised control trial based on two geographic sites	Quasi-experimental, non-randomised design
Results	Decreased hospital inpatient and nursing home use; increased utilisation of outpatient medical care, therapies and home- and community-based services; positive impact on Medicare costs vis-à-vis non-enrolee comparison group; favourable health status outcomes; overall satisfaction with care arrangements; inconsistent impact on physical functioning; differences in quality of life (not statistically significant)	Increased access to home- and community-based services; reduced hospitalisation of alternate level of care patients (i.e. 'bed blockers'); decreased utilisation and costs of emergency department, hospital inpatient and nursing home stays (not statistically significant); average community care costs per person were higher in SIPA group, but institutional costs were lower with no difference in total overall costs per person in two groups; no differences in health outcomes; increased satisfaction for SIPA caregivers with no increase in caregiver burden or out-of-pocket costs	Declining trend in institutionalisation and client preference to be institutionalised; no deterioration in autonomy/functioning at T1 and T2, but effect disappeared at T3; little effect on utilisation of services; positive effect on carer burden; no impact on mortality (survival)

the transformative impact of integrated care, greater attention should also be focused on client- or user-defined outcomes (see, e.g., Beresford and Branfield, 2006; see also Chapter 11). To be successful, not only whole system models must prove that they do a better job of managing services and costs than the disjointed systems of health and social care they are intended to replace, but they should also demonstrate ultimate acceptance and satisfaction by the consumer. Although this chapter has drawn on a series of North American models, these remaining challenges seem important issues for all health and social care systems to reflect upon and seek to resolve.

Summary

- The frail elderly present a complex set of multifaceted needs which demand a comprehensive, coordinated package of long-term care services to maintain independent living in the community for as long as possible.
- In order to improve long-term care continuity, effectiveness and efficiency, a number of developed countries are experimenting with whole system models of partnership working that more or less tie together an array of health and social services for the frail elderly under one organisational roof.
- North America has become a fertile proving ground for these integrated service arrangements. Three well-known models are PACE in the US and both SIPA and PRISMA in Canada.
- Evaluations of the successful PACE, SIPA and PRISMA programmes point to a promising pattern of outcomes in terms of measures such as access, clinical coordination and continuity, level of functioning, service utilisation, institutionalisation, carer burden, client satisfaction and costs.
- Several common programmatic ingredients appear to explain the positive results of the three integrated care prototypes analysed: (1) umbrella organisational structure; (2) case-managed, multidisciplinary team care; (3) organised provider network; and (4) financial incentives (at least in the case of PACE).
- Although these results travel in the right direction, the experiences of PACE, SIPA and PRISMA also suggest that models such as these are still 'works in progress', and the effective integration of long-term health and social care through the means of a single organisational structure can be a complicated and difficult undertaking.
- Despite the extensive evaluations involved in these projects, much more work needs to be done in order to understand the explicit relationships between structures, team working arrangements, service delivery and outcomes in integrated service models.
- Since the ultimate test of a new service approach is consumer acceptance and satisfaction, future research must also do a better job of focusing on client- and user-defined outcomes.

Further reading and useful websites

For an earlier discussion of integrated care for the frail elderly in the American context and a detailed comparison between the PACE and the Social Health Maintenance Organisation models, see:
Kodner, D. and Kay Kyriacou, C. (2000) Fully integrated care for the frail elderly: two American models, *International Journal of Integrated Care*. Available online via http://www.ijic.org

For a review of US, Canadian, Italian and Australian models of integrated care for frail older persons, see:
Kodner, D. (2002) The quest for integrated systems of care for frail older persons, *Aging Clinical and Experimental Research*, 14(4), 307–313.

For a wide range of interesting articles on various aspects of systems of care for the frail elderly from a global perspective, see:
Bergman, H. and Béland, F. (eds) (2002) *Aging Clinical and Experimental Research*, 14 (Special Issue on Systems of Care, 4), 223–318.

For a discussion of various forms of long-term care integration that have been developed in Denmark, Germany, the Netherlands, and Sweden, see:
Kodner, D. (2003) Long-term care integration in four European countries: a review, in J. Brodsy, J. Habib and M.J. Hirschfeld (eds) *Key Policy Issues in Long-Term Care*. Geneva, World Health Organisation (WHO). Available online via http://www.who.int/chp/knowledge/publications/policy_issues_ltc/en/index.html

For an historical and policy perspective on so-called managed long-term care programmes in the US, see:
Saucier, P., Burwell, B. and Gerst, K. (2005) *The Past, Present and Future of Managed Long-Term Care*. Washington: DC, Department of Health and Human Services, Office of Disability, Aging and Long-Term Care (ODALTC). Available online via http://aspe.hhs.gov/daltcp/reports/mltc.pdf

A rich collection of international articles and reviews on various forms of integrated care can be found in the *International Journal of Integrated Care*: http://www.ijic.org

Information on the PACE model, its evaluation and recent developments can be found on two websites:
The National PACE Association website: http://www.npaonline.org/website
The Medicare website: http://www.medicare.gov/Nursing/Alternatives/Pace.asp

Additional information and updates on the SIPA and PRISMA models can be found on two websites:
Studies and data on the SIPA programme are found on the website of Solidage, the Research Group on Integrated Services for Older Persons co-sponsored by the University of Montreal and McGill University: http://www.solidage.ca/e/sipa/htm
Studies and updates concerning the PRISMA programme can be found at the website of the Program of Research on Integration of Services for the Maintenance of Autonomy: https://www.prismaquebec.ca/cgi-cs/cs.waframe.index?lang=2

References

Ansak, M. (1990) The On-Lok model: consolidating care and financing, *Generations*, (Spring), 73–74.

Béland, F. *et al.* (2006) A system of integrated care for older persons with disabilities in Canada: results from a randomized control trial, *Journal of Gerontology: Medical Sciences*, 61, 367–373.

Beresford, P. and Branfield, F. (2006) Developing inclusive partnerships: user-defined outcomes, networking and knowledge – a case study, *Health and Social Care in the Community*, 14(5), 436–444.

Bergman, H. *et al.* (1997) Care for Canada's frail elderly population: fragmentation or integration, *Canadian Medical Association Journal*, 157, 1116–1121.

Bergman, H. *et al.* (2003) Evaluation of a system of integrated care (SIPA) in Montréal, Quebec, Canada: a 22-month randomised control trial with 1230 frail older persons, *Journal of the American Geriatrics Society*, 51 (4, Suppl.), 532.

Bodenheimer, T. (1999) Long-term care for frail older people: the On Lok model, *New England Journal of Medicine*, 341, 1324–1328.

Chatterji, P. *et al.* (1998) *Evaluation of the Program of All-Inclusive Care for the Elderly (PACE): The Impact of PACE on Participant Outcomes*. Contract No. 500-96-0003/TO4. Baltimore, US Health Care Financing Administration.

Dowling, B., Powell, M. and Glendinning, C. (2004) Conceptualising successful partnerships, *Health and Social Care in the Community*, 12(4), 309–317.

Eng, C. *et al.* (1997) Program of all-inclusive care for the elderly (PACE): an innovative model of integrated geriatric care and financing, *Journal of the American Geriatrics Society*, 45, 223–232.

Feder, J., Komisar, H. and Niefeld, M. (2000) Long-term care in the United States: an overview, *Health Policy*, 19, 40–56.

Glasby, J. and Littlechild, R. (2004) *The Health and Social Care Divide: The Experiences of Older People*, 2nd edn. Bristol, Policy Press.

Glasby, J. and Peck, E. (eds) (2003) *Care Trusts: Partnership Working in Action*. Abingdon, Radcliffe Medical Press.

Hébert, R. *et al.* (2003) PRISMA: a new model of integrated service delivery for frail older people in Canada, *International Journal of Integrated Care*. Available online via http://www.ijic.org

Hébert, R., Tourigny, A. and Gagnon, M. (2005) *Integrated Service Delivery to Ensure Persons' Functional Autonomy*. Montreal, EDISEM.

Hollander, M. *et al.* (2002) *The Cost-Effectiveness and Cost-Benefit of Home and Community Care within the Broader Continuum of the Health System*. Report Prepared for Home and Continuing Care Unit, Health Services Division, Health Canada. Victoria, Hollander Analytical Services Ltd.

Hudson, B. *et al.* (2002) *Executive Summary 26: National Evaluation of the Use of Section 31 Partnership Flexibilities of the Health Care Act of 1999*. Manchester/Leeds, National Primary Care Research and Development Centre, University of Manchester/Nuffield Institute for Health, University of Leeds.

Jacobzone, S. (1999) *Ageing and Care for Frail Elderly Persons: An Overview of International Perspectives*. Labour Market and Social Papers No. 38. Paris, Organisation for Economic Co-operation and Development (OECD).

Johri, M., Béland, F. and Bergman, H. (2003) International experiments in integrated care for the elderly: a synthesis of the evidence, *International Journal of Geriatric Psychiatry*, 18, 222–225.

Kane, R., Illston, L. and Miller, N. (1992) Qualitative analysis of the program of all-inclusive care for the elderly (PACE), *The Gerontologist*, 32, 771–780.

Kodner, D. (2002) The quest for integrated systems of care for frail older persons, *Aging Clinical and Experimental Research*, 14(4), 307–313.

Kodner, D. (2003) Long-term care integration in four European countries: a review, in J. Brodsky, J. Habib and M. Hirschfeld (eds) *Key Policy Issues in Long-term Care*. Geneva, World Health Organisation.

Kodner, D. (2004) Beyond care management: the logic and promise of vertically integrated systems of care for the frail elderly, in M. Knapp *et al.* (eds) *Long-term Care: Matching Resources to Needs*. Ashgate, Aldershot.

Kodner, D. and Kay Kyriacou, C. (2000) Fully integrated care for the frail elderly: two American models, *International Journal of Integrated Care*. Available online via http://www.ijic.org

Kodner, D.L. and Spreeuwenberg, C. (2002) Integrated care: meaning, logic, applications, and implications – a discussion paper. *International Journal of Integrated Care*, 2. Available online via http://www.ijic.org

Leutz, W. (2005) Reflections on integrating medical and social care: five laws revisited, *Journal of Integrated Care*, 13(5), 3–11.

National PACE Association (2005a) *PACE Programs Around the Country*. Available online via http://www.npaonline.org/website/article.asp?id=71

National PACE Association (2005b) *Who Does PACE Serve?* Available online via http://www.npaonline.org/website/article.asp?id=50

OECD (2005) *Long-Term Care for Older People*. Paris, Organisation for Economic Co-operation and Development.

Tourigny, A. *et al.* (2004) Evaluation of the effectiveness of an integrated service delivery network (ISD) for the frail elderly, *Canadian Journal on Aging*, 23(3), 231–245.

Trahan, L. and Caris, P. (2002) The system of care and services for frail older people in Canada and Quebec, *Aging Clinical and Experimental Research*, 14(4), 226–232.

White A.J. (1998) *Evaluation of the Program of All-Inclusive Care of the Elderly (PACE) Demonstration. The Effect of PACE on Costs to Medicare: A Comparison of Medicare Capitation Rates to Projected Costs in the Absence of PACE*. Contract No. 500-96-0003/TO4. Baltimore, MD, US Health Care Financing Administration.

WHO and Milbank Memorial Fund (2000) *Towards an International Consensus on Policy for Long-Term Care of the Ageing*. Geneva, World Health Organisation.

Zimmerman, Y., Pemberton, D. and Thomas, L. (1998) *Evaluation of the Program of All-Inclusive Care for the Elderly (PACE): Factors Contributing to Care Management and Decision-Making in the PACE Model*. Contract No. 500-96-003/TO4. Baltimore, MD, US Health Care Financing Administration.

6 Working across the health and social care boundary

Amanda Edwards

As several chapters in this collection suggest, understanding *how* to manage relationships across organisational and professional boundaries has received less attention than analysis of the difficulties and barriers to effective coordination between policy makers, service commissioners and providers and practitioners. Recognition and analysis of these problems is important, but it is arguable that the *how* is perhaps even more significant. This chapter sets out to answer two specific questions. Firstly, what is it necessary to do to ensure that these difficult, cross-boundary relationships are well managed and enhance the delivery of services and experience of people who use services? Secondly, given that this is a problem common to the organisation and delivery of services for older people across the developed world, what can be learnt from the experience of a number of different countries? Along with the chapters by Henk Nies (Chapter 4) and by Edward Peck and Helen Dickinson (Chapter 1), this should aid students and practitioners to better address the 'how' factor of health and social care partnerships.

This chapter aims to explore the nature of relationships that can sustain cross-boundary work and argues that particular actions or behaviours (e.g. establishing a philosophical base and providing a funding mandate) create the conditions in which those tasked with the responsibility can work across boundaries more effectively. Box 6.1 briefly describes the research on which this chapter is based. The chapter then introduces a conceptual framework (the tripod of work) for the analysis of working relationships, and examines research evidence through this lens, highlighting critical features at particular boundaries: between government departments; between acute and community services (at transition); between local service providers; and between central and regional levels of government (at implementation). It concludes with a summary of key points and implications for managing working relationships at the boundaries between health, housing and social care.

The tripod of work

The challenge of creating a conceptual framework for the analysis and comparison of the evidence from research in countries with significantly different ways

---

Box 6.1   The research.

This chapter is based on research undertaken for an MPhil thesis (Edwards, 2003) which provides an international comparison of different ways of managing boundaries in the care of older people. In the care of older people, there are multiple boundaries between social care, housing and health:

- Within and between organisations
- Between different levels of government
- Between professions and disciplines

A literature review on coordination and policy implementation (which identified critical environmental factors, benefits, difficulties and potential flaws in effectively managing boundaries) was supplemented by empirical research in a range of countries. The countries selected for the research (Germany, Denmark, Australia, the Netherlands, the US and Italy; see Table 6.1 for further detail of programmes in these countries) were chosen as purposive case studies, rather than as a representative sample, in order to provide contrasts in philosophy, constitutional structure and in the way services are funded and organised. The case study methodology adopted for this study follows that outlined in Schulz and Greenly (1995). According to this approach, data are gathered and analysed using a conceptual framework (in this case the tripod of work; see below for further discussion). During the course of the research, over one hundred forty people were interviewed who worked in a wide range of service and policy settings, including national, state/regional and local government, and in a variety of service providers, all of whom were doing similar jobs or tasks in the countries (e.g. assistant secretary in the Department of Health and Aged Care, Australia, and the equivalent position in the Federal Ministry for Health, Germany; team leaders of an elder care programme in Wisconsin, USA, and of a municipal domiciliary and nursing service in Horsens, Denmark).

---

of organising services for older people is considerable. This research made extensive use of the work of Gillian Stamp and colleagues at Bioss (Brunel Institute for Organisational Studies) (see, e.g., Saunders, 1997; Stamp, 1999), whose tripod of work (see Figure 6.1) provides an analytical framework for probing how boundaries are managed in practice. It is highly empirical, based on conversations with people being led and managed, and has been used in practice in different cultures and organisations in many parts of the world. The Bioss tripod works from the premise that it is the nature and quality of working relationships that are crucial to the success of an organisation. This is then further refined to address the nature of the external relationships that an organisation must create, sustain and make effective in order to operate successfully. The tripod describes three qualities which are essential to create working relationships that add value: *judgement, coherence* and

Table 6.1 Key features of case study programmes.

Programme	Country	Key features
Cross-boundary policy work		
Integration of housing and long-term care	Denmark	Clear parameters were set and resources allocated accordingly. Responsibility and finance for housing for older people was transferred to the Ministry of Housing, and the legislation provided for both new schemes and the refurbishment of old institutions. One organisation became responsible within each district for home care in people's own homes, nursing homes and staffed units, plus home nursing and equipment and adaptations.
The acute/community boundary		
Transition care pilots	Australia	Aged care assessment teams put together a funded package of interim support for people following discharge from hospital
Martin Luther Stiftung and Hanau Hospital rehabilitation services	Germany	Collaboration between local hospital (which refers and provides clinical supervision) and a care provider (which provides accommodation and personal care). Also provides 24-hour cover for people who receive care at home
Homeward 2000	Australia	Collaboration between a domiciliary care provider, local general practitioners and a local hospital, which aims to prevent admission to hospital
Horsens Hospital and municipality – hospital discharge agreement	Denmark	Regular review of quality; municipality nurses visit patients before discharge and provide continuity between primary and secondary care
Managing implementation		
Case management schemes	America/ Australia	Teams are accountable for working with service users to find the best possible solutions. Teams operate to a spending limit per person on the programme to set up a package of care specifically designed to an individual's needs with considerable flexibility to purchase services
Boundaries between providers		
Lapham Park assisted living	US	A public/private partnership between six organisations to provide coordinated health, housing and social services to support older, low-income adults to live at home
Cape Cod Health Care – care continuum	US	The Cape Cod Health Care continuum (two hospitals, physicians' practices, home nursing, the hospice and laboratory services) has developed care maps for the management of various illnesses
Care network – Bologna	Italy	Provides a single source of referral and is the means through which case managers coordinate care and arrange, for example, outpatient appointments, home dentistry as well as home help or day care
Silver Chain Care	Australia	Nurses, personal carers and home helps are all members of the same team, which assesses and provides nursing and personal care
Horsens municipality domiciliary service	Denmark	A nurse leads the team of assistant nurses and home helps. While the nurse undertakes specialist care, home helps assist with personal care tasks, administer medication as directed by the nurses and do housework

Trusting: maintaining vigilance

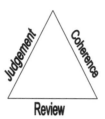

Tasking: Tending:
facing transactional dilemmas   preserving the relationships

Figure 6.1 The tripod of work – working across organisational boundaries. (Source: Stamp, 1999.)

review. These qualities are underpinned and sustained by three activities: *tending*, *trusting* and *tasking*. The remainder of this section outlines these aspects in more detail and they are used to structure the presentation of data in the remainder of the chapter.

Clear *tasking* helps to avoid the tendencies of all parties to look for swift, individual gain and negotiate and bargain to achieve a win for their own side – rather than focus on the joint objective. Tasking is described as the first step towards realising the mutual interests of the relationship and involves:

- sharing intention and agreeing objectives;
- anticipating transaction costs;
- considering and evaluating other ways of undertaking the task;
- creating parameters by agreeing the end product, a target time for completion and resources (time, authority, budget, etc.).

Such precision, it is argued, creates 'safe' conditions in which to proceed and allows for review without blame. In contrast, *tending* is the more invisible task of keeping things working in a way which keeps people and purposes aligned (keeping people on board) and includes:

- agreeing how disputes will be resolved;
- nurturing and establishing the tone of the relationship;
- making sure systems are in place to support the work and that relevant information is available.

Vigilant *trust* is not a soft fuzzy feeling; its vigilance lies in the fact that it is neither distrustful nor unquestioning. It considers both the interests of cross-boundary work and the reputation of the participating organisations and maintains clarity so that those involved are not overwhelmed by the ambiguities or complexities of the project. A key relationship across organisational boundaries where vigilant trust has been supported by tasking and sustained by tending will, the model suggests, develop the following qualities:

- The parties will share a *coherent* understanding of the purpose and goals of the project and the relationship – they will know what they are there to do and why (and this view will be held in common).
- They will feel empowered to use their *judgement* to take forward the mutual interests of the relationship.
- There will be an in-built capacity to *review* progress, use resources efficiently and address (and remedy) problems.

The user's perspective

The acid test of how well (or otherwise) boundaries are managed lies in the perceptions and experience of people who use services. There is strong evidence that people want providers to join up services for them rather than having – to stretch a metaphor – to sew the seams themselves (Edwards, 2007; for an alternative view, see Chapter 10). People find health and social care systems confusing; there is frustration at having to repeat the same personal information to many different people and at the lack of good information about services. In a paper on older people's definitions of quality services, Qureshi and Henwood (2000) identify staff competence and continuity of care and of staff as two important features of quality services (others include flexibility, reliability and having sufficient time). Continuity emerges as a particularly important factor for the oldest older people – those likely to have the highest needs for assistance. This suggests that when boundaries are managed effectively this should result in:

- *easier access to services*, either because there are fewer points of entry to the service system or because staff know the system and can refer on with confidence;
- *fewer assessments*, or ones which build on the previous assessments so that people do not have to repeat their story;
- some *continuity of staff* coming into the home;
- *choice* about where to live.

Alongside the tripod of work, this list provides another lens through which to examine the effectiveness of cross-boundary work. Moreover, this perspective is based on what partnership working should achieve in terms of service user outcomes – whereas the tripod might be said to refer to organisational outcomes.

It is often a long journey from the development of a policy to a change in practice or service delivery which may result in, for example, less duplication or greater continuity for users. Previous research has been criticised (e.g. Webb, 1991; Waldvogel, 1997) for tending to look at only one level, for example, concentrating on just policy development or service delivery. This chapter follows various stages of this journey, starting with cross-boundary (or joined-up) policy development and finishing with a case study service area (in this case, domiciliary care).

Cross-boundary work at the centre

Both Waldvogel (1997) and Fine *et al.* (1998) note that better working across boundaries is as important at government level as it is at the level of service delivery. However, Pollitt observes what a difficult task joined-up government is between government departments (Pollitt, unpublished). In this study, a number of countries had made efforts to tackle the boundary between housing and care in this way. For example, in Denmark the 1987 reforms saw the start of a joint approach which was backed by a common philosophy that emphasised independence, integration and empowerment. Responsibility and finance for housing for older people was transferred to the Ministry of Housing, and the legislation provided for both new schemes and the refurbishment of old institutions. One organisation became responsible within each district for home care in people's own homes, nursing homes and staffed units, plus home nursing and equipment and adaptations. In the 1990s a further subsidy stimulated development of, for example, specialised living groups for people with dementia, which enabled people to live in their own accommodation (with a tenancy) with specialist support.

The coordinated model of policy making found in Denmark demonstrates many features of the tripod of vigilant trust. The aims were clear and the intention (that people would retain maximum possible independence in their own home, with the provision of care no longer linked to the dwelling) shared. It was clear from conversations with officials that a shared philosophical base had been significant in setting the tone and sustaining the relationship over time – even when personnel changed. Clear tasking and the establishment of vigilant trust meant that those involved could use judgement to take (or recommend) decisions (e.g. the transfer of responsibilities from two ministries to one). This was in the interest of the overall project, but represented a loss of resource (and control) for one party. When confronted by difficulties (such as gaps in the level of service for people with dementia), tasking and tending had created the capacity to review and then make changes within the framework of the new philosophy and structure of provision. More recent changes to the fees structure, which again required close interdepartmental work, show a continuation of shared intent (ensuring coherence) and clear decision-making. Such clarity has lessened the transaction costs, with some duplication being abolished at the start and the clear allocation of responsibilities decreasing the chance of disputes about funding.

Waldvogel (1997) and Leutz (1999) both outline the importance of funding in supporting desired policy changes. In Denmark a shared philosophical base created a framework of intent that has been sustained over time and supported by funding changes. In the Netherlands a shift in funding to allow the use of residential and nursing care budgets for outreach services for people with a needs assessment for 24-hour care was important in stimulating cross-boundary work. Discussions about joint policy development with policy makers – whether it concerned rural policy, hospital discharge or housing – gave rise to interesting insights into barriers encountered and what is significant in helping people to work better together. These included the importance of clear objectives, of an ability to spot opportunities to advance both your own and other departments' policies, and of a willingness to sit through and work with disagreements.

The prevention of impoverishment in old age is an explicit aim of German long-term care policy in line with a commitment to social solidarity. Clarity of focus (what are we aiming to change, do differently and why), of objectives (which are agreed), and setting up the task properly with adequate support and agreed timescales emerge as significant to making things work, along with the ability to solve and work with problems and pay attention to the process as well as the task. Frustration arises when people feel that this type of work is seen as marginal, an activity in which others are unwilling to engage. This adds to the picture beginning to emerge of what helps work between and within government departments. Tasking seems to be particularly important, with considerable emphasis on clear, shared objectives: a mandate to work together – which is strengthened by a shared philosophical base.

The acute/community boundary: managing transition

All the countries involved in the research are challenged to some degree by the boundary between acute and community care and the necessity to make this bound-ary function more effectively. Hospital discharge and the development of rehabil-itation have been identified in all these areas as problematic. The main reasons for this are that responsibility and, therefore, funding for acute and community ser-vices lie either at different levels of government or (as in Germany) with separate parts of the insurance system. Responses to this issue (as described in Table 6.1) range from making coordination across this boundary a specific task to creating some budget flexibility and stimulating joint local approaches. In all of the exam-ples, a clear mandate from the funders had been important. Insurance funds in Germany are keen to shorten length of stay in hospital and their attitude was seen as an important factor in the development of rehabilitative services. In Denmark, legislation and guidance set a framework for improving the management of this boundary. In these cases emphasis was also put on tending relationships. As earlier outlined, tending is the activity which takes account of inevitable uncertainty and anticipates problems. It facilitates the development of agreements and protocols which characterise the management of this boundary.

In Horsens, staff commented that the hospital discharge agreement generally works well. However, they have to work at the relationship and problems do still occur in terms of insufficient notice and unrealistic care plans – particularly if the patient is not known to the service. Time spent working with hospital staff had paid off and means when things go wrong they can deal with. This had recently led to a very honest review and discussion of the quality of hospital notes. However, this is not easy, and anxiety about the acute sector's demand on resources and the consequent need to protect community services has therefore to be taken into account in the way that the acute/community boundary is managed. Many of the examples rely on good multidisciplinary teamwork, demonstrating – it could be argued – vigilant trust in action. Acute and community services have much to protect, both organisationally and professionally. In the examples given the task is clear, with local players understanding what is intended, but with some freedom to use their discretion about how to achieve this. Funding is available and attention paid to keeping relationships going. The results show an ability to use judgement within the limits agreed for the work and with accountability for both shared and separate goals. Vigilant trust means that although the work is difficult, those involved are sufficiently mandated and supported to work effectively together.

The national/regional boundary – managing implementation

Some boundaries benefit from being tightly drawn whilst others do not; getting the right balance can be critical for successful implementation. The way that assessment is used in all the countries in this research suggests that decisions about the level of benefit need to be quite tightly managed (although not too prescriptively, as this runs the risk of excluding people). However, this applies much less when it comes to decisions about what services should be provided when greater flexibility in provision and improved continuity can be achieved. Australia and Germany use classification systems to allocate long-term care, whilst in America classification is used for reimbursement with the same intention. In all three countries, criticism had been made that tight classification based on tasks and direct care does not readily take account of the care needs of people with dementia. Reforms have tackled this in Australia, and in Germany the matter was being taken up by the Länder (state governments). In the US, the state of Wisconsin is addressing this as requiring skilled nursing in assessment for support to meet long-term care needs by including medication, monitoring and behaviour management.

This comparison provides a good example of managing the boundary between policy and practice. All of these methods are designed to ensure clarity, fairness and to control the allocation of resources. Too much specification can limit discretion and innovation and, paradoxically, exclude needy groups (dementia being a case in point). Setting the task has become more like giving instructions, with the result that it is over-specified, and the results for users (lack of responsiveness to changing need) are clear. On the other hand, too little clarity is confusing both for users and for those who have to implement these policies. Case management schemes in the US (Wisconsin) and Australia bring together staff from different professional backgrounds. Both schemes operate within fixed budgets and within criteria that govern eligibility for the scheme. Teams find the ability to innovate exciting and feel both challenged and supported to do this:

> I've never been unable to do something. (Care Manager, Madison, WI, USA)

As a result, some innovative solutions to people's problems have been found:

> When people are telling stories about what they have thought to do, everyone gets excited. (Manager, Community Options Programme, Perth, Australia)

Both managers and evaluators from the University of Wisconsin observed benefits for users in terms of:

- better care plans – as people debate and learn from each other;
- better practice – as nurses adopt a more participatory approach, social workers' knowledge of medical conditions improves.

However, purchasing flexibility is accompanied by quite tight management of the financial boundary. At the level of implementation, there is a degree of prescription, which sets the parameters for the exercise of discretion in practice. It is this clarity, combined with the sharing of expertise and freedom to use the budget, which seems to produce innovation and quality improvement.

Some boundaries benefit from being more tightly drawn. A clear distinction between funding for housing and funding for care is made in Australia, the Netherlands and Denmark. (This same distinction is also maintained in charging for nursing and residential care in Germany.) As one commentator in Copenhagen (Denmark), commented, '[I]t is a paradox that we separated housing and care to get to the right place'. To achieve this, a very clear distinction was made between the responsibility for providing housing and for providing care so that, unlike institutional care, support is no longer linked to the dwelling. People would retain the maximum possible independence in their own home, with the level of care being assessed and provided according to their particular need. The replacement of nursing and residential care with a combination of specialist housing and a joint local nursing and domiciliary care service has led to the development of assisted living models. People retain their own accommodation and financial responsibility for it, with support services (which also provide care to the surrounding area) based in the building. For users the great advantage is being able to remain in the accommodation of their choice because it is suitable and because the right level of care is available.

A similar model is found in the Netherlands. The funding and provision of care and housing is kept separate. There is some chafing at what are perceived to be unnecessary restrictions, but such a clear boundary does create greater flexibility. The Australian, Dutch and Danish models mean that support can be provided to people as and when they need it, without it being tied to accommodation. Schemes funded under the Supported Accommodation Programme in Victoria (Australia) manage a set number of cases in state housing. When a housing allocation is made, the programme provides the necessary level of support. Only once minimal support is required does the agency takes on a new case, for whom a home is allocated from the housing waiting list.

The message is clear that tight management of the housing and care boundary at a policy level can produce greater flexibility. Access to services is more straightforward and people have a choice about where they live. The boundary between policy and implementation and practice is being managed in a way that sets the framework, but does not prescribe the detail. It would seem that in the management of the housing and care boundary, clarity about funding streams and roles enables people to trust and use their judgement and initiative. Tending is demonstrated in the attention paid to the way in which changes are managed and the setting up of systems and procedures to support this. The evaluation of schemes, establishment of working arrangements between housing and social services, ring fencing of resources and the specification for accessibility are all examples of practical steps to nurture and preserve relationships. Thus, the coherent understanding of the task is translated into new types of services.

Working across boundaries between providers

It is important to note that coordination may not always be the answer to complexity. In a review of the literature, Fine *et al.* (1998) find that there is no one single approach which can provide solutions to the problems of service fragmentation in community care. Instead, they propose that the concepts applied to different degrees of collaboration form a scale or continuum, which extends from autonomy to integration, to distinguish between the various types of activity across organisational boundaries (this is similar to the depth–breadth axis outlined in the Introduction to this book and to Leutz's concepts of linkage, coordination and integration in Chapter 3):

- *Autonomy* is when agencies act without reference to each other, although their actions may affect one another.
- *Cooperation* is when parties show a willingness to work together with an emphasis on communication.
- *Coordination* is when considerable effort is put into harmonising the activities of agencies so that duplication is minimised. This is often characterised by the activity of a third party to coordinate and the existence of agreed protocols.
- *Integration* is when the boundaries begin to dissolve and new work units emerge.

The countries studied in the research provide some examples of cooperation (see Table 6.2), which, supported by tasking and tending, can produce good results for users from joint working between organisations. The examples show that when the right conditions are created through effective tasking (such as the sharing of common purpose, supported by a funding mandate, which was described at Lapham Park, Cape Cod and Hanau) and tending to sustain motivation and collaborative teamwork, well-directed cooperation can bring some positive results for users. A willingness to work together, supported by good communication, is all characteristic of cooperation (Fine, 1998). Moreover, in these cases it is suggested that these examples demonstrate effective joint working between partners. For example, the Lapham Park project has improved access to services and enabled residents to age in place. Networks in Bologna and the Cape Cod Care Continuum show a similar pattern – with significant discussion between autonomous agencies to achieve more efficient referrals and less duplication.

These examples also show the importance of tasking through levels of implementation and service delivery by providing a policy and funding mandate. This can

Table 6.2 Key messages.

Programme	Country	Key messages
Transition care pilots	Australia	There was a clear mandate from funders,
Martin Luther Stiftung and Hanau Hospital rehabilitation services	Germany	combined with some flexibility about the use of budgets
Homeward 2000	Australia	Time and attention paid to key relationships is a
Horsens Hospital and municipality	Denmark	critical factor in managing relationships at the acute/community boundary
Integration of housing	Denmark	A shared philosophical base underpinned the clear mandate, funding changes and tight management of the housing and care boundary that drove the development of the policy
Case management schemes	America, Australia	Prescribed spending limits, combined with flexible purchasing and a loosening of professional boundaries, create conditions for the exercise of judgement and innovation
Lapham Park	US	Cooperation between autonomous, local agencies,
Cape Cod Health Care	US	within a framework of a clear shared purpose
24-hour service, Hanau	Germany	and focused effort to sustain innovation and
Care networks, Bologna	Italy	teamwork, can bring some positive results for users
Silver Chain Care	Australia	Good supervision and flexible team roles can
Horsens municipality	Denmark	enhance quality and continuity of service

be in the form of a 'fit' with the prevailing policy environment, a shift in funding, increased scrutiny and mutual benefit, aiding the sharing of intent and discovery of areas of common interest. The project at Hanau is consistent with a drive to shorten length of stay and improve aftercare. This aids the establishment of mutual benefit, particularly where funding is concerned. Lapham Park benefited from a shift in housing practice: federal funding is pushing a more coordinated approach. This is a major change for housing staff who are used to an exclusive focus on bricks and mortar: as one provider in Milwaukee, Wisconsin, said, 'it all fell into place at the right time'. Knowing that HMOs (see Chapters 3 and 5 for further detail) will scrutinise and spot duplication is one incentive to work better together. In Cape Cod the development of a continuum of care plan, in which agencies agree on how care for particular conditions should be managed, was partly a result of pressure from funders to reduce duplication and costs.

But what about the level of direct contact with service users? All the providers involved in the research saw continuity for users as very important and approached this by adopting a team model of working. Both Horsens and Silver Chain show how new types of jobs are beginning to emerge as tasks are shared or allocated more flexibly with appropriate supervision. The nature of team working provides the right conditions for this, enabling home care workers to use their judgement but with accountability. Both teams stress the importance of supervision to maintain quality. Locally based services and knowing all the members of teams also contribute to greater continuity for individuals. There is realism about the limits, though – that is, recovering at home from a stroke will mean a lot of staff visiting (but the aim is they should explain their purpose) and both the models described have different day and night arrangements. This does raise the question of how much continuity is possible. The literature on service user's views (e.g. Farrell *et al.*, 1999; Qureshi, 1999) distinguishes between two sets of activities, which, from the service user's perspective, improve continuity. One is the same people visiting (and this applies particularly to the provision of personal care); the second is the proper exchange of information between professionals so there is some continuity of action and purpose.

Conclusion

Across government the sharing of intent through a shared philosophical base is important to underpin coordinated policy development in challenging areas. In Denmark a strong commitment to citizenship and to the independence of older people, which was shared between the ministries of housing and social affairs, informs past and current policy developments, resulting in the provision of assisted living for older people. A shared philosophical base is also a feature of Germany's implementation of their long-term care insurance.

Leutz (1999) argues that the level of integration should be defined by the circumstance, taking into account such factors as stability, urgency, severity and duration of the condition (see also Chapter 3). Management of transition appears to be one of the defining factors with a need for coordination, supported by a mandate from funders to develop the necessary protocols and desired changes in practice. Cooperation, through joint working supported by effective tending, tasking and trusting, can secure good results for users. Key messages from each of the programmes about what is important in managing boundaries are outlined in Table 6.2.

The lens of the tripod has thrown additional light on when relationships need to be loose and when to be tight, showing that tight parameters at a policy level that set a clear framework for implementation are helpful, but that the tendency to stray into detail has to be watched. Policy can helpfully prescribe roles and responsibilities (particularly between housing and care) and the framework for the allocation of benefit or resources. At a more local level of implementation, funding parameters combined with purchasing flexibility work well. The message is simple: be clear but do not over-specify at the macro level.

Finally, there do seem to be some clear benefits to service users from the team models that a number of providers discussed in this chapter have developed. For service users, greater continuity of staff and the combination of nursing supervision with domiciliary care stand out. A threat to this is low status (and pay), high turnover and, in some places, great difficulty in recruitment. One way suggested of tackling recruitment problems is to create a career path for people who provide 'flexible care' which crosses the health/social care boundary. Some of the ways in which staff skills are combined in the team approaches described in this chapter suggest there could be considerable benefits to this.

Summary

- A shared philosophical base, which underpins policy, can be significant in securing changes to policy, service delivery and practice.
- Anxiety about the acute sector's demand on resources (and the consequent need to protect community services) recurs as a theme of managing the acute/community boundary.
- The factors that help manage transitions at this boundary include a mandate from funders, agreement about which resources are shared and which are protected, clear parameters for the work and careful attention to key relationships.
- Policy and implementation should aim for a careful balance between prescription and discretion so that systems are seen to operate fairly, yet can respond to individual need and encourage innovation.
- Separating the responsibility for housing and care (so that care is not linked to accommodation) enables innovative schemes where intensive help is provided whilst preserving people's autonomy.
- There are clear benefits from integrated team working in the provision of community-based home, domiciliary and nursing care in securing continuity and improved management of chronic illness and disability in old age.
- Designing jobs which cross the nursing/home care boundary could achieve greater continuity for people. It would also provide an opportunity to develop workforce skills and improve career development.

Further reading and useful websites

Useful texts include:
Fine, M., Thomson, C. and Graham, S. (1998) *Evaluation of New South Wales Demonstration Projects in Integrated Community Care*. Sydney, Social Policy Research Centre, University of New South Wales.
Glendinning, C. (ed.) (1999) *Rights and Realities: Comparing New Developments in Long-Term Care for Older People*. Bristol, Policy Press.
Nuffield Institute Community Care Division (2000) *A Partnership Assessment Tool*. Leeds, Nuffield Institute.
Schulz, R. and Greenly, J. (eds) (1995) *Innovating in Community Mental Health – International Perspectives*. New York, Praeger.
Trompenaars, F. and Hampden Turner, C. (1997) *Riding the Waves of Culture: Understanding Cultural Diversity in Business*. London, Nicholas Brearley Publishing.
Waldvogel, J. (1997) The new wave of service integration, *Social Service Review*, (September), 463–484.

Relevant websites include:

http://www.silverchain.org.au

http://www.humanitas.nu (Dutch only, but English coming soon)

http://www.geroinst.dk

http://www.carewisc.org

http://www.academyhealth.org/2003/presentations/broadhead.pdf (presentation by Peter Broadhead on *Government Initiatives in Coordinated Care: Australia, UK and US – Testing the water or swimming the Channel?*)

http://www.kda.de/ (German only)

http://www.bioss.com

References

Edwards, A. (2003) *Look for What You Can Do, Not for What You Cannot.* Unpublished MPhil thesis, Leicester.

Edwards, A. (2007) Partnership working and outcomes – a case of the hare and the tortoise? *Journal of Integrated Care*, 15(1), 24–26.

Farrell, C., Robinson, J. and Fletcher, P. (1999) *A New Era for Community Care? What People Want from Health, Housing and Social Care Services.* London, Kings Fund.

Fine, M., Thomson, C. and Graham, S. (1998) *Evaluation of New South Wales Demonstration Projects in Integrated Community Care.* Sydney, Social Policy Research Centre, University of New South Wales.

Leutz, W. (1999) Five laws for integrating medical and social services: lessons from the US and UK, *Millbank Quarterly*, 77(1), 77–109.

Qureshi, H. (1999) Outcomes of social care for adults: attitudes towards collecting outcome information in practice, *Health and Social Care in the Community*, 7, 257–265.

Qureshi, H. and Henwood, M. (2000) *Older People's Definitions of Quality Services.* York, Joseph Rowntree Foundation.

Saunders, A. (1997) *Leadership and Optimal Organisation of Work: The Power of the Tripod.* London, Bioss.

Schulz, R. and Greenly, J. (eds) (1995) *Innovating in Community Mental Health – International Perspectives.* New York, Praeger.

Stamp, G. (1999) *Working Together.* London, Bioss.

Waldvogel, J. (1997) The new wave of service integration, *Social Service Review*, (September), 463–484.

7 Partnerships in the digital age

Justin Keen and Tracy Denby

Markets in health and social care have dominated policy making around the world for a long time, but policy makers know they cannot live without partnerships. The same apparently compelling logic is employed in many countries. Partnerships involving health, social care and other organisations continue to be problematic. In the face of inexorable forces (principally demography and technological advances), services are becoming ever more complex and ever more expensive. Against this background, it is often argued that the only efficient way of addressing these challenges is through partnership working. There is only one policy option: redouble efforts to improve the effectiveness of partnerships. And now we have electronic networks which, by their nature, are ideal technologies for linking people and organisations; they will help in our quest for more effective partnership working this time round.

This chapter examines the claim that networked electronic services are essential to more effective partnership working. In the next section we set out an idealised model for the delivery of integrated electronic services, and in subsequent sections use the model to aid judgements about the extent to which electronic services support partnership working at the moment and the directions in which information technology policies are taking us. The final section looks forward setting out two possible futures, one approximating to our idealised model and the other to a more mundane outcome, where new services serve only to reinforce existing professional and organisational contours. We present contributory evidence from our own research that hints at which future seems more likely at the moment.

The aspiration

Many readers would have seen references in the media to something called Web 2.0, and moved swiftly on. After all, the Web is a synonym for geek, and it sounds dangerously close to the stuff that the spotty guy at school was doing. In practice, though, Web 2.0 is concerned with some important phenomena that seem set to affect us all. Anyone familiar with Second Life or with social networking services such as MySpace and Facebook will know that it is easy to create a personal space for sharing information. Like riding a bike, anyone can do it. The best services can handle any type of data, including photos and videos, and have their own email services. (Indeed, reports from Hitwise show that the use of MySpace webmail has been growing so fast that it is responsible for a marked *decline* in Hotmail and other web-based email use.) These services can be used in either of two ways. In one, the aim is to maximise the number of 'friends' who have access to your space: organisations such as the Fabian Society welcome friends to their Facebook service. Anyone can post papers, contribute to online discussions, advertise forthcoming events and so on. In the other, the aim is to create a secure space where you retain control over your friends. You are happy for friends to see photos of your children, or to discuss plans for the party next weekend, but you do not want the whole world to see them.

These services are already used by millions of people around the world, and it does not seem too fanciful to aspire to similar services focusing on health and social care, where we can interact with our various care providers. Yet the contrast with the state of information technologies in most health and social care organisations could hardly be starker. While many health and social care professionals and administrators use information technologies routinely in their jobs, the vast majority of systems are 'stand-alone'. That is, systems have been developed over the last two decades around the needs of individual general practitioners (GPs), individual hospital departments and to support specific social services functions. They have not been designed to support the sharing of personal data, and it turns out that there are significant barriers in the way of linking these systems together. The major exception is email and internet access, but most people have access these days, and it would be more remarkable if staff did not already use them.

The task, then, is to move from stand-alone to integrated services. If we take the social networking analogy at face value, each of us citizens should have our own space in a service – we could call it Careweb – and we would give permission for carers and others to access our space. It would be very easy to set up, and would be able to handle any data – medical notes, X-rays, the outcome of your care assessments and so on. It would include the ability for people to mail one another or post general queries to the people managing your care. The permissions would change over time, and we would be able to control those permissions. The logic of social networking also suggests that Careweb would not be limited to the boundaries of current health and social care delivery, but would include informal support, ranging from a friend nearby to an online support group.

Given the ubiquity of social networking services and the fact that Web 2.0 has been foreshadowed for many years, one might be forgiven for assuming that information technology policies around the world are focusing on creating Carewebs. In practice, a few commercial companies promote a model along these lines, providing secure environments for patients to maintain their own health and health care data, but as we will see governments are pursuing very different policies. This suggests that we need to investigate two issues. The first is the gap between aspiration and current realities on the ground, and the second is the gap between the idealised model and the policies being pursued by many governments.

Organisational realities and policy responses

Looking at the realities on the ground first, other chapters demonstrate that public services are still too often poorly coordinated. Separate government departments continue to work in 'silos' with equally separate policy communities. Commissioning of services has historically tended to be along functional lines, with health and social care commissioning only now beginning to come together. We need look no further to understand why so many health and social care staff are still using stand-alone computer systems: systems developers have merely acted in the same way as everyone else and worked with the grain of existing functional divisions.

Equally, there has been a growing realisation that complex social problems cannot be tackled within traditional silos. Whether services are organised in hierarchies or in markets, there needs to be coordination of resource allocation and service delivery. Indeed as Hood (2005) points out, coordination is a classical problem in public administration, and whatever terms are used, the various policies are all variations on the theme of promoting effective coordination.

What are the policy responses to these coordination problems? Policies designed to promote partnership working generally acknowledge that it is a challenge, and this holds across countries with very different institutional structures such as England, the Netherlands, Australia, Canada and the USA (Kickert *et al.*, 1997; Lewis, 2006). The term *partnership* is still widely used, but in recent times similar policies have been presented under the banners of 'whole systems' working, networks and care pathways. An example concerning managed local networks for children's services in England illustrates two problems relevant to electronic services:

> Managed local networks differ from other types of partnerships in that they have clear governance and accountability. For example, integrated service arrangements may already be 'managed local networks' as long as they have governance and accountability arrangements in place. For many managed local networks these arrangements may need to be linked to those for one or more children's trusts. Managed local networks are therefore defined as: A linked group of health professionals and organizations from primary, secondary and tertiary care, and social care and other services working together in a coordinated manner, with clear governance and accountability arrangements. (Department of Health, 2005, p. 11)

The first problem is that readers will search in vain for any details about the claimed accountability arrangements. Indeed, the reason why children's services are network-like – rather than, say, system-like or examples of partnerships – is never explained. Figure 7.1 usefully captures the quality of policy thinking; we are invited to think of networks as squiggles joined by slightly unsteady lines. The second, and unsurprisingly, policies that promote networks do not contain any clues about the way in which the government thinks that electronic services will make the joined-up squiggles more effective. It is difficult to imagine how any serious computer scientist could get from Figure 7.1 to a proper understanding of the kind of electronic service that would support the members of any network.

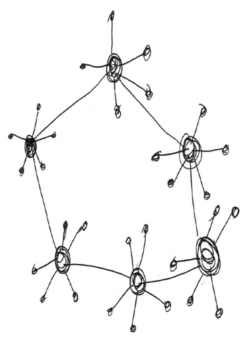

Figure 7.1 Department of Health depiction of a network of children's services. (From Department of Health, 2005, p. 9.)

If partnership (and whole system and network) policies are vague about the nature and role of electronic services, what of information technology policies? It turns out that the news is not good here either. The central assumption driving investments in many countries is that the infrastructure of large-scale information technologies and the services that run over them represent good investments (Tang, 2002; Spil *et al.*, 2004; Keen, 2006). In England, for example, information technologies have been given a prominent role in pursuit of 'information age government through IT'. The government argued that IT would 'make it much easier for different parts of government to work in partnership', as well as, 'help government to become a learning organization by improving our access to, and organization of, information' (Prime Minister and Minister for the Cabinet Office, 1999, Chapter 5, para 5). This point is worth emphasising: governments are persuaded that *integrated* electronic solutions will be cost-effective.

In passing, we should stress that governments are not investing on the basis of evidence, although this is not entirely their fault. The majority of the empirical evidence, drawn from studies across Europe and north America, focuses on stand-alone systems, reported in the health services research literature and else-where (Delpierre *et al.*, 2004; Poissant *et al.*, 2005). Conversely, there are social science journals devoted to the study of information technologies in health and other contexts, but in all bar a few cases the literature focuses on high-level accounts of the implementation and use of systems and services. The same could be said of the information systems, management and political science literatures (see Galliers *et al.*, 2006). By their nature, these literatures offer few clues about the value of information technologies in supporting partnerships, or indeed into any causal mechanisms that may be involved.

Fortunately, the absence of empirical evidence does not prevent us from continuing with our analysis. If we look at the technologies that governments favour – and policies are similar in many countries – then some general patterns are visible. There are two main types of services. The first is communication, exemplified by specific services such as the electronic transfer of prescribing information between GPs and pharmacies, and the use of email for general purposes. The second is access to single personal records, including health and social care records. The presumption appears to be that the two will support better partnership working. It will come as little surprise by now to hear that policies fail to specify exactly how, or in what contexts, these services will improve partnerships.

The reasons may not be hard to find. In practice, these policies are generally being pursued either by governments or by large firms (such as insurance firms operating in insurance-based health care systems), and policy documents make it clear that they have other purposes in mind. Viewed from the top of an organisation, part of the attraction of it lies in continuous monitoring of everyone's work. (Indeed, the same is true lower down – many systems are sold partly on the promise of enabling managers to monitor and evaluate front-line staff.) Large-scale electronic networks can therefore have a strong tendency towards central control built into them.

So, modern networked services can have major political tensions built into them. On the one hand, they may support 'horizontal' partnerships in both commissioning and service delivery. On the other hand, networks are typically funded and controlled by states or by top management teams in private or social insurance bodies, and they may well be interested in 'vertical' control. This latter use, or even the potential for that use, makes them less attractive to some users, and the medical profession in particular has consistently objected to plans for large-scale networks over many years.

Seen in this light, current UK 'transformational government' (Cabinet Office, 2005) policies look distinctly double-edged. The government claims that the quality of public services will be improved if individual departments can share data. The claim is apparently straightforward, namely that departments need to coordinate their activities, so as to provide more integrated and person-centred services, and in order to do this they need to share data about individuals. In England the legislative framework, driven in part by beliefs about terrorism, is making it easier over time for the state to access and use personal data. A benign interpretation here is that there will always be tension between integration and personal data protection (6 *et al.*, 2006). In contrast, commenting on a report that he had commissioned, the information commissioner warned that we may be sleepwalking towards a surveillance society (see Surveillance Studies Network, 2006). Transformational government policies, and perhaps large-scale networks in general, may lead to perverse interpretations of partnership working. The partnerships in mind are those between the state and its various agencies, rather than horizontal partnerships focused on service users.

Two futures: fractured or integrated?

Given the arguments to this point, it may seem perverse to suggest that we need to think about the role of information technologies in partnership working in the future. If the past is any guide at all, the future is clear and it is fragmented at the level of commissioning and provision, and worryingly integrated at the level of the state. There are, though, two plausible reasons to consider where we may be heading. The first is that there are signs that the general environment is changing, and the prospects for partnership working may be more propitious. It would be naïve to be too optimistic, but the emphasis appears to be moving away from market-based thinking back to partnerships and other joined-up government policies (Dunleavy et al., 2006). The second reason, and perhaps the more compelling, stems from our earlier observations about social networking. Even though it is stretching credulity in one direction to argue that partnerships will be much more successful in the future, it is stretching it in the other direction to suggest that something like Carewebs will never happen. New internet-based services are everywhere, are cheap and easy to use, and eventually someone will come along with a service that everyone likes.

To make progress we need a simple framework for thinking about the ways in which electronic services do – or might in principle – support partnerships. Here we use concepts drawn from public administration and socio-legal studies (Hood, 1998; Sabel, 2004). Imagine, for a moment, that five people need to be involved in the treatment and care of Mrs K: two work in the NHS, one in social services, one for a voluntary organisation and one for a private provider. The details of Mrs K's needs do not matter particularly, but perhaps she is an older person with some health problems, living on her own with children nearby. Many writers on partnership would take the view that there are two main types of partnership here, one between Mrs K and the five care providers, and the other among the care providers, who need to coordinate their actions with one another.

Fractured – the new public management scenario

How likely is it, then, that Mrs K will be supported by a team using her Careweb? One interpretation of current patterns of use of electronic services is that they will tend to reinforce existing professional and organisational relationships. They will strengthen the loose ties that bind professionals together across time and space to use Castells' (2001) phrase.

Following Dunleavy and Margetts (2000) and Braithwaite and Drahos (2000), we believe it is useful to think of health care systems as networks of 'political nodes', where nodes are places that are occupied and controlled by professional or other groups. If the future develops along the lines of new public management style changes of the past, then the emphasis will be on competition and control. GPs substantially control what happens in their practices, social workers and their teams and so on. The control of many of the nodes in health and social care systems is long established. Of course, the control is not absolute, but change will not occur unless the key people are persuaded.

Electronic services lead to competition for nodes. Viewed this way, there is a long-standing competition for ownership of electronic patient records. During the 1990s, policy documents in many countries fudged the issue of ownership of such records (which at the time existed in very few places): ownership lay somewhere between the managers who paid for them and the clinicians who used them in their work. (There was no serious lobby in favour of patients or clients owning their records.) Currently, the competition for both ownership of medical records (in essence the legal right to say who has access to them) and the day-to-day control over them (which more commentators now believe should be shared between service providers and patients/clients) is ongoing. The advent of electronic personal medical records therefore seems set to intensify competition.

There is a related but distinct competition for the ownership and control of information about patients and clinicians themselves. There is a promise/threat (depending on your point of view) that information technologies will be used to performance manage clinical work. Not altogether surprisingly, doctors and other professionals have not generally responded well to these suggestions. It does not seem surprising that professionals have either commandeered information technologies for their own use or resisted attempts to (as they see it) impose them. In this scenario, Mrs K's needs seem likely to get lost in the turf wars between the various parties and in the centripetal pull of the state, acting as a global performance manager. The future need not be entirely bleak, if Mrs K's carers can find ways of working together on the ground, shielding themselves from the excesses of events above them. But the value of a Careweb will be directly related to the extent to which local staff are willing and able to work together.

Integrated – digital era governance scenario

In Abbott's (1988) attractive metaphor, professional groups change over time, both internally and in relation to one another, in the same way that tectonic plates rub against one another and change shape over millenia. The landscape alters when relationships between professional groups alter. Dunleavy and colleagues (2006) argue that just such a tectonic shift is occurring in public services around the world, driven in significant part by the ubiquity of the internet and other information technologies. They term this shift 'digital era governance': it is slowly but surely replacing new public management as a basis for policy thinking and is characterised by some of its opposites, particularly in the desire to promote 'joined-up' solutions and to provide person-centred services. Neither of these latter concepts is at all new – the argument is that after years of exhortation, these policy ideas are (finally) central to policy thinking, due in part to the tendency of networked technologies to place them there.

This second future is the one where Careweb becomes a more realistic possibility. The precepts of *Modernising Government* (Prime Minister and Minister for the Cabinet Office, 1999) have – due more to technology than good policy making – seeped into working practices. Social scientists tend to be sceptical about technological determinism, but in this scenario the availability of technology, combined with enthusiastic uptake by some service users and some service providers, leads to subtle but real pressures on others to follow suit. Mrs K may or may not control her own space – its ownership may be fudged and just sit somewhere between the main users. For us the main point is that Careweb is part and parcel of a move towards partnership working, at least among Mrs K's carers.

The future may lie somewhere between the two scenarios and indeed may vary from country to country. The key point is that there are claims on Mrs K's space. Commissioners want access to summary data, to help plan care for Mrs K and the rest of the local population. Mrs K might control her own space in some countries, but not in others. In more 'individualistic' societies, service users are already owners of their own records – they carry medical records from one doctor to another. And Mrs K's views of her own space may also depend on the nature of the support she needs. If she has a long-term condition, for example, she may wish to coordinate her own care. Conversely, she may have little interest if she feels her health problems are temporary in nature.

Some evidence: diabetes care

Which scenario is more likely? Some evidence from our own research may shed a little light on the question. An exploratory study has been undertaken to investigate the implications of an integrated electronic health record used in the management and treatment of diabetes. The findings provide some evidence of the ways in which electronic services can support partnerships between health and care services, thereby enhancing patient care and management. The system (called SystmOne) is employed within Airedale Primary Care Trust and Airedale General Hospital (further details of the system may be found at the end of chapter). It provides a comprehensive service, not entirely unlike Careweb, but with the crucial difference that it is clear that the system is owned by the local NHS, not by any patient or local resident. This was not Mrs K's service. The service allows for the sharing of information between a wide range of health care professionals. Medical records include all consultations, drug issues, patient and doctor communications, and pathology results. It is also possible to attach documents through scanning. And it has its own 'notification' system – roughly the equivalent of a mail service in social networking sites such as Facebook. Because data are updated constantly and accessible instantaneously, all health care professionals involved in the care of a patient can share information in real time. Since diabetes patients are likely to receive care from a range of clinicians and health professionals, the integrated record has the potential benefit of preventing problems associated with conflicting information, duplicate tests and procedures.

Detailed observations of the service in use provided insights into the different ways in which it was being used in clinical encounters, the circumstances where it had effects on clinical practice and the ways it was being used as a form of communication. Three broad conclusions were drawn from the evidence. Firstly, the integrated record had greatest impact on supporting partnerships at the primary–secondary interface. Secondly, there were settings in which an integrated record service would have limited impact on patient care and management. Thirdly, the potential benefits were influenced by the extent to which health care professionals used it as a means of communication.

Where both secondary and primary care staff used SystmOne, there was clear evidence that using the system allowed for better patient management by enabling access to the whole patient record. Diabetes consultants within secondary care, for example, would use the record to familiarise themselves with patients' circumstances prior to a consultation, to see how they were being managed within primary care, whether they had seen other specialists, their recent blood test results and current medications. If a patient was not, however, registered at a general practice that used SystmOne, the record was used much less by the consultant, as it would not have been updated since the previous outpatient appointment. The lack of a shared service resulted in the consultant spending a significant proportion of the appointment time gathering patient histories, particularly about medication. Limited information sometimes prevented consultants from altering the medication of a patient, instead referring a patient back to his or her GP. Within primary care, diabetes specialist nurses spoke of the advantages of having a shared electronic record that allowed them to monitor a patient's recent health care treatment and management. It was, for example, apparent if a patient had not attended an appointment with other services, such as the renal or ophthalmic services.

Whilst the majority of health care professionals involved in the care of diabetic patients benefited from being able to access an integrated record, there were certain contexts in which having access to a complete medical record was not as essential as others. For example, podiatrists working in the foot clinic rarely referred to a patient's record, due to both their familiarity with patients who they saw on a regular basis and the nature of their work. Sometimes, records are just not integral to patient care.

SystmOne has a secure internal messaging service. This attribute allows health care staff to send and receive confidential information about patients, share the record, send and receive messages from any SystmOne user as well as be alerted to new pathology results. Communicating to a wide range of health care professionals using this feature was widely regarded, by staff, as a potentially effective and efficient way of managing the treatment and care of diabetic patients, particularly across the primary–secondary care interface. Evidence revealed this to be under-utilised, however, principally because not every health care professional involved in the care of diabetes patients used SystmOne. Some staff also felt they had not had sufficient training to use the facility. There was, therefore, a lack of confidence with the system. Staff could not be certain that 'notifications' would be read. There was still a belief that using the phone or fax was a superior way of ensuring that something urgent was dealt with. Indeed, referrals to other health care services were not made within SystmOne and actively discouraged by some departments within secondary care. Paper referrals were still used in both primary and secondary care. It became apparent that different communication strategies were appropriate according to the setting. Since specialist services were located within close proximity within the diabetes centre at the hospital, face-to-face discussion between colleagues was an effective means of communication regarding patient management.

The study has enabled us to begin to build a picture of the different ways in which the service is used in clinical encounters and how it may support partnerships between health care professionals and different services. In terms of our two broad scenarios, the evidence appears to point in both directions. The fact that the service is used across primary, secondary and specialist services suggests that the digital era governance scenario is not completely far-fetched. The comment that key staff were not using the service is important. Several specialties at the hospital are not using the service, even though it has been used within diabetes for several years. Digital era governance has some way to go before it becomes a reality across all services, even in that locality. As we have already observed, we are a long way off integrated services across whole regions or countries. Countries such as Denmark, where they do have integrated electronic services (Danish Centre for Health Telematics), are the exceptions that prove the general rule.

Conclusion

Whatever the future holds, it seems that electronic services are likely to play a greater role in the organisation and delivery of health and social care. Progress towards integration may continue to be hampered by well-established political problems, or the promised 'transformation' may be more likely than sceptical academics realise. Either way, one of the casualties may be the partnership concept itself. If things continue to go badly, partnership will once again be cast out and other policy prescriptions sought. But if things go well, will we still have partnerships? If even part of the Careweb idea is realised, it will support dynamic relationships among a number of partners. While one might call these relationships partnerships, the digital era brings with it two other words that may better describe what is happening – network and system. As we have seen, policy makers' grasp of these two terms is, if anything, even less solid than it is of partnerships, but our attention may nevertheless switch to these broader, more nuanced concepts.

Summary

- The technology now exists to allow individuals to own and control their health and social care records and selectively permit care providers access to those records.
- Information systems will not necessarily promote better coordination of care: they are not a 'magic bullet' for promoting partnership working.
- Governments around the world tend to be more concerned with accessing data about the volume and quality of services than promoting individual ownership of care records. The risk of 'sleepwalking towards a surveillance society' is real in some countries.
- The quality of policy thinking about the role of information systems is disappointing. It seems likely that information systems will both help and hinder partnership working in the future, but there is scant evidence that policy makers anywhere are thinking seriously about their effects.

Further reading and relevant websites

Useful sources include:

Dunleavy, P. *et al.* (2006) *Digital Era Governance: IT Corporations, the State, and e-government.* Oxford, Oxford University Press.

Hanseth, O. and Ciborra, C. (eds) (2007) *Risk, Complexity and ICT.* Cheltenham, Edward Elgar.

Relevant websites include major ongoing IT programmes such as the following:

Details of SystmOne: http://www.tpp-uk.com/marketing/casestudies.html and the research study at http://www.sdo.lshtm.ac.uk/cpehealth.html

The NHS National Programme for IT: http://www.connectingforhealth.nhs.uk

The Danish Centre for Health Telematics: http://cfstuk.temp.fyns-amt.dk/wm150976

References

Abbott, A. (1988) *The System of Professions.* Chicago, University of Chicago Press.

Braithwaite, J. and Drahos, P. (2000) *Global Business Regulation.* Cambridge, Cambridge University Press.

Cabinet Office (2005) *Transformational Government: Enabled by Technology.* London, Cabinet Office.

Castells, M. (2001) *The Internet Galaxy.* Oxford, Oxford University Press.

Danish Centre for Health Telematics. Available online via http://cfstuk.temp.fyns-amt.dk/wm150976

Delpierre, C. *et al.* (2004) A systematic review of computer-based patient record systems and quality of care: more randomized clinical trials or a broader approach? *International Journal of Quality in Health Care*, 16, 407–416.

Department of Health (2005) *A Guide to Promote a Shared Understanding of the Benefits of Managed Local Networks*. London, Department of Health.

Dunleavy, P. *et al.* (2006) *Digital Era Governance: IT Corporations, the State, and e-government.* Oxford, Oxford University Press.

Dunleavy, P. and Margetts, H. (2000) *The Advent of Digital Government: Public Bureaucracies and the State in the Internet Age.* Available online via http://www.governmentontheweb. org

Galliers, R., Markus, M. and Newell, S. (eds) (2006) *Exploring Information Systems Research Approaches: Readings and Reflections.* London, Routledge.

Hitwise: Available online via http://www.hitwise.com/resources/whitepapers-and-reports.php

Hood, C. (1998) *The Art of the State.* Oxford, Oxford University Press.

Hood, C. (2005) *The Idea of Joined-Up Government.* Oxford, Oxford University Press.

Keen, J. (2006) Information technologies: so beguiling, so difficult, in K. Walshe and J. Smith (eds) *Healthcare Management.* Maidenhead, Open University Press.

Kickert, W., Klijn, E.-H. and Koppenjam, J. (eds) (1997) *Managing Complex Networks: Strategies for the Public Sector.* London, Sage.

Lewis, J. (2006) *Health Policy and Politics: Networks, Ideas and Power.* East Hawthorn, Australia, IP Communications.

Poissant, L. *et al.* (2005) The impact of electronic health records on time efficiency of physicians and nurses: a systematic review, *Journal of the American Medical Informatics Association*, 12, 505–516.

Prime Minister and Minister for the Cabinet Office (1999) *Modernising Government.* London, The Stationery Office.

Sabel, C. (2004) Ungoverned production, in J. Gordon and M. Roe (eds) *Convergence and Persistence in Corporate Governance.* Cambridge, Cambridge University Press.

6, P. *et al.* (2006) Partnership and privacy – tension or settlement? The case of adult mental health services, *Social Policy and Society*, 5, 237–248.

Spil, T. *et al.* (2004) Electronic prescription systems: do the professionals use it? *International Journal of Healthcare Technology and Management*, 6, 32–55.

Surveillance Studies Network (2006) *A Report on the Surveillance Society.* Report for the Information Commissioner. Available online via http://www.ico.gov.uk/upload/documents/library/data_protection/practical_application/surveillance_society_full_report_2006.pdf

Tang, P. (2002) AMIA advocates national health information system in fight against national health threats, *Journal of the American Medical Informatics Association*, 9, 202–203.

8 The economics of integrated care

Marie-Eve Joël and Helen Dickinson

This chapter explores and analyses how in economic and financial terms, 'integrated health care networks' for older persons and people with chronic or complex conditions are organised. In order to understand different types of financing, we will look at a number of examples of networks across the world and examine the relation between funding methods used and how networks function. Despite the growing importance of this task, this is a far from simple process (as will be demonstrated below).

The chapter starts with a brief note on the nature of networks and terminology before going on to consider some of the various forms and funding arrangements networks in the international arena have taken. We then examine the evidence of cost-effectiveness for these networks and summarise key themes regarding the finance of integrated care networks. Some of these discussions overlap at the margins with those of other chapters (such as those by Dennis Kodner and Helen Dickinson, Chapters 5 and 11). Although the focus of this chapter is on economics, some discussion of form and evaluation is necessary in presenting a complete perspective on this issue.

Networks and a note on terminology

Health care networks first began to develop in the international arena in the 1980s. Although many of these tended to be informal to begin with, they have often developed to take on recognised legal frameworks and in a number of areas have been granted public funding. In the 1990s they became more widespread, encompassing different pathologies and different population groups. At the same time, systematically analysing these networks became a major issue in a context where health and welfare policy is increasingly subject to financial constraints (Dominiak *et al.*, 2006). Many integrated health care networks developed in response to problems encountered by systems of long-term care for older and frail people. Two prominent issues which were drivers of these developments (and which were outlined in detail in the Introduction to this book) are the following:

1. *The increasing complexity and fragmentation of health and social care systems.* This fragmentation poses particular difficulties in information exchange, meaning

professionals do not always have access to the data needed to improve the overall functioning of the network. Consequently, expensive services (e.g. hospital accident and emergency) are used inappropriately and there can be long waiting lists for certain services.

2. *Growth in demand for long-term care and the total cost of such care.* The long-term health care sector is dealing with a massive increase in individualised patient care (in light of ageing populations and new pathologies). Current funding methods tend to be either heterogeneous, focused on the medical profession with well-defined rights on the one hand, or dependent on the social security system and often much more precarious on the other.

In response to these pressures some decision-makers, administrators and health care professionals suggest that the 'network' embodies a certain ideal of economic perfection. It is seen as combining the knowledge of professionals in providing care in a way that is as rational as possible and offers the best value for money. At this point it is worth noting that although in this chapter we refer to networks, there is no one 'essence' of network and these exist in a variety of forms. Each of these forms has its own definition of integrated care, funding structures and are known by many terms – for example, managed care, intermediate care, transmural care, seamless care, person-centred care and chain of care (Leichsenring, 2007). All these forms exist at different points on the depth–breadth axis outlined in the Introduction (Figure 2). The values which tend to be associated with integrated care networks include individualised care, coordinated care provided by a multidisciplinary team, individualised follow-up care for frail older people and, more generally, higher standards of care. This chapter examines different notions of networks in order to determine whether their funding systems are indeed neutral in terms of cost or whether they are intended to influence the behaviour of those involved in the network to encourage the process of integration into the network – that is, whether such mechanisms are capable of providing efficiency savings and simultaneously more effective and patient-centred services.

Different network funding models

Different types of funding may be classified according to the underpinning purpose of the network. The economic and financial incentives brought into play in the network increase according to the extent of network integration. Here we make the distinction between:

- public funding for good practice;
- funding coordinated health care programmes;
- funding totally integrated health care networks.

Public funding for good practice

In this simple financial model, network operating costs and related services for vulnerable people included in the network are directly funded by public authorities without this affecting the financial architecture of the health care system. In other words, it is suggested that by working together in a network, health and social care services are able to provide better targeted patient care, thus saving at least as much money on the hospital system or treatment in medical/welfare institutions as that spent on running the network. Funding is often provided for a limited period and under experimental conditions. The implicit hypothesis is that this will reveal areas of inefficient spending that can be restructured by coordinating those involved. However, as suggested by Esterman and Ben-Tovim (2002) from a series of Australian studies, the opposite may also be true. That is, a lack of coordination may hide a lack of resources, implying that the development of a coordinated network will reveal needs that are not met, thus potentially not saving any money at all (at least in the short term).

Supposing that the system is financially neutral or, if one prefers, generates a minimal return on investment, it is proposed that it is then possible to reproduce this kind of experimental network. Those involved in the network are not given any strong, direct economic incentives to alter behaviours but are subject to post hoc financial assessments. Examples of this are the gerontological networks in France (57 out of the 458 were publicly funded networks). These have succeeded the '*Soubie*' networks, which were the first general networks with a structured framework. These networks negotiate budgets with the regional authority for a period of 3 years, but there is little specificity about the form they must take. Furthermore, these networks are able to waive certain French social security rules and have access to special funding (experimenting with new ways of paying health care providers and the contributions of patients with social security cover, etc.).

This first model implies a need for a minimum level of cost accountability, with transparent accounting and no hidden costs, that is, a free contribution to running the network from one of the organisations that hosts it (which, for example, provides personnel or keeps the network accounts).

Funding coordinated health care programmes

A coordinated programme is a structure or procedure common to all the partners involved set up to provide a better response to the complex and changing needs of frail people, for example, a single treatment centre with a case manager. Each participant in the network retains his or her own organisational base, but adapts it to take part in what Hébert *et al.* (2003) calls 'an umbrella system'. There are a number of examples of such models we will consider here (some of which are mentioned in other chapters): the Darlington project, PRISMA (Programme of Research to Integrate Services for the Maintenance of Autonomy) and PRISMA France.

The English Darlington project, 1985–1986 (Challis *et al.*, 1991, 2006), used a case management approach to manage an alternative to hospitalisation for people requiring long-term care. The case manager had a total budget for the 20 people under his or her care, calculated on the basis of two thirds of the cost of institutional care (average cost of a bed for a prolonged hospital stay). The case manager's financial action was totally central to the model and operates on two levels. Firstly, the response to the older person's needs proposed by the case manager was developed in line with budget restraints and with a view to direct cost control. Secondly, the budget provision enabled the case manager to get involved in network management and in integrating professionals from all the different services in the network. In this case the NHS funded the experiment (i.e. the job of the case manager). The point of note with this model is not the way it is funded, but the use of a management approach within a multidisciplinary team in an attempt to reduce overall costs.

A second, more complex, example of coordination is the Canadian PRISMA model (see Chapter 5 for more detail of this book). The research project attached to this model was primarily interested in assessing the set up and impact of integrated health care networks. The programme was backed by substantial public funding from all the public actors involved. An experiment is now underway to try and set up PRISMA in France at three experimental sites (Somme et al., 2007). The funding agreed by the State and Social Security office is intended solely for research in support of the experiment. No additional budget is forthcoming for the experimental sites themselves.

Funding totally integrated health care networks

'Totally integrated' health care networks take full responsibility for all the services offered to a population within an area, within the framework of a single organisation (Leutz, 1999; see also Chapter 3). One of the objectives of this is to achieve the highest level of flexibility in satisfying demand. We consider three different examples here:

- Integrated networks in which the financial mechanism is central (e.g. On Lok, PACE, Social HMO and SIPA). Pooling resources through capitation funding is a major means of saving money used by these networks.
- Integrated networks without an integrating financial mechanism but with very dense human resources management (e.g. two Italian networks developed in Rovereto and Vittorio Veneto).
- Last, we will look briefly at the French Ancrage network (a cross between PRISMA and SIPA).

Several major programmes in the US, such as On Lok/PACE and Social HMO (again, see Chapter 5 for further detail on these programmes), have opted for capitation funding (i.e. where funding is limited at a certain amount on the basis of an enrolled population, rather than on a fee-for-service basis). The On Lok project was reproduced at several sites under the PACE programme (Program of All-Inclusive Care for the Elderly) (Eng et al., 1997), while the Canadian CHOICE programme (Comprehensive Home Option of Integrated Care for the Elderly) aims to allow frail population groups to be cared for at home as part of a vast programme that includes care for acute illness as well as long-term care and social services. Integration is achieved insofar as the offer of services and personnel is based on the concept of financial integration. For On Lok/PACE, funding came from Medicare, Medicaid and private contributions from patients included in the network but who were not eligible for Medicaid. Medicaid's contribution was a percentage of the amount paid by each state for the care of a comparable frail population (varying from 1 to 4, depending on the state concerned). Medicare's contribution was based on the AAPCC (average area per capita cost) multiplied by a 'vulnerability' adjustment factor negotiated with the administration that funds health care (2.39 in 1995). In such conditions, revenue through capitation varies widely from one site to another. This mode of funding provides greater flexibility in allocating resources and in spending, without restricting the use of resources. The programme has full control over all long-term health care spending and covers all the financial risks related to health care, including for the frail population. This provides a strong incentive for preventive care and rehabilitation (Lee et al., 1998).

The Social HMO programme is a project funded at federal level, which combines the services provided by Medicare with a modest range of long-term care services. It targets older people in general, not only frail older people. The desired result is to redirect some of the money spent on acute care for frail patients to long-term care, and the programme therefore includes a social services component. The funding method is the same as that used for PACE (Kane et al., 1997). The difference between the two models lies in the fact that the vulnerability factor is applied to all the members of the network under PACE, whereas under the Social HMO the programme restricts the number of people included who are potentially eligible for long-term care and sets a threshold on the volume of home services (Kodner and Kyriacou, 2000).

SIPA (Système Intégré pour les Personnes Âgées fragiles) draws inspiration from the On Lok/PACE model. This is a system of integrated health care and social services which is responsible for elderly frail people within a given area and which uses case management and a per capita prepayment system. Its specific feature is that the issue of funding is central to the system. Flexible use and rapid mobilisation of resources are the conditions required to ensure that the network functions effectively. The underlying idea is that the financial fragmentation of a fragmented network is a cause of inefficient use of resources. The idea is to transfer the cost of institutional services to local services, thereby cutting the use of institutional services (i.e. less recourse to emergency services, reducing the length of hospital stays, cuts in permanent residential care, reducing the amount of time spent in hospital waiting to be placed in a nursing home) and making more intensive use of local services. Total costs remain the same and there is no transfer of the cost of care to the elderly or to their informal caregivers. In a second phase of the SIPA project, the plan is to set up a capitation funding scheme and extend this during a third phase.

The Rovereto and Vittorio Veneto models in Italy are intended to organise continuity and coordination of care from the geriatric ward to the home, with a single point of entry to the network (Bernabei et al., 1998; Landi et al., 1999). The case manager provides support to the general practitioner (GP), helping the latter to integrate into the multidisciplinary team. The idea is that the GP should be closely involved in care management, which may produce positive impacts without it being necessary to include a financial incentive for the substitution of services in the network. The GP is not dispossessed, unlike some other networks where the patient cannot choose his or her own GP, and maintains full clinical responsibility for the situation. The case manager coordinates care, supported by the geriatric assessment that is the starting point for everyone in the network, but without having a specific budget. Family resources are used in exactly the same way in the control group and in the group taking part in the experiment.

The Ancrage network (DeStampa *et al.*, 2007) in France has operated since October 2006 and offers a model that combines elements of SIPA and PRISMA. It performs assessments, develops care plans and provides follow-up care for around one hundred frail elderly people recruited through a central office. These patients are selected on the basis of age, dependency and isolation. Care is provided by the network partners coordinated by the case manager (hospitals, home help services, local information and coordination committees, GPs, etc.). Regional public funding covers network operating costs (fees for the geriatric specialist and the case manager). Two specific points are worth noting here:

- The case manager performs two kinds of task: dealing with long-term follow-up care for a large number of patients and managing emergency situations for a smaller number of patients.
- The network is structured in response to failures in the provision of care identified by health care professionals.

Cost-efficiency assessments

Drawing on examples of cost-efficiency assessments of networks for long-term care, this section aims to examine whether it is possible to demonstrate that different forms of network financing are cost-effective. On the whole, integrated care systems for frail older people that rely on home care services tend to produce good results from the perspective that they adapt care to patient needs and reduce institutional treatment and costs. Whether the network is cost-effective or not is intricately linked to the health care system Johri *et al.*, 2003), and the combination of case manager, in-depth geriatric assessment and multidisciplinary team appears to be a key to success in this respect. In fact, the existence of a multidisciplinary team is proposed to ensure that the geriatric assessment will be followed up with effective action, that frail people receive the services they need and, therefore, that the offer of services will be managed appropriately (Johri *et al.*, 2003). In this section we analyse the economic aspects of these assessments in more detail (and readers may also find Chapter 11 useful in considering the outcomes of some of these programmes in more detail).

French gerontological networks

The French General Inspectorate of Social Affairs (Daniel *et al.*, 2006) carried out a review of public funding for all health care networks in France. Its analysis was highly critical: French evaluations were limited to examining the structure of the network set-up and an appreciation of how the project developed. They did not produce any reliable indicators of the results on clinical, management or financial levels: 'There was little to learn from the assessments. They were very few in number, the methodology used was very heavy and the interpretations are disputable. Unit costs were rarely assessed, even summarily' (Daniel *et al.*, 2006, p. 3).

The only national assessments made concerned the experimental *'Soubie'* networks in 2003 and 2005, the results of which suggest the following:

- The death rate of patients cared for through the network was lower and the total number of trips to emergency departments was reduced.
- The savings made attributed to the network were in terms of hospital spending, offset operating costs and the costs of related services (check-ups and follow-up of network patients). Outpatient spending was considered to be exactly the same within or outside the network, even though structured differently. Transport costs are higher in the network while outpatient, medicines and physiotherapy spending are slightly lower.

The study concluded that in the case of publicly funded networks in France, there is no rigorous analysis assessing the cost-effectiveness of integrated health care networks for frail people. The difficulties in developing such assessments include the following:

- The networks' bureaucratic administrative procedures.
- The lack of unified accounting follow-up in a context where the number of various coordinated care services for the elderly has substantially increased (local information and coordination committees, integrated health care networks, coordinated care centred around the local hospital, etc.)
- The absence of clear assessment objectives defined for the networks by the publicly funding authorities.

Coordinated care networks

The culture of analysing these forms has developed to a much greater extent in English-speaking countries. A more or less experimental, non-random model with a control group of institutionalised patients (Challis *et al.*, 1991) suggested that the costs of the Darlington network were much lower, taking costs as including not only the cost of services but also the time needed for patient assessment and working out/setting up care plans. Savings were made in all the scenarios thanks to a substantial reduction in the amount of time spent in health care institutions, although there were some reservations regarding the patients selected for the assessment (Challis *et al.*, 1991).

The PRISMA evaluation reported that older people cared for in this network had more autonomy and higher satisfaction rates, although death and institutionalisation rates were not affected. However, there were less emergency services used and hospitalisation rates and costs tended to be stable. Total costs remained constant as did spending on care for older people. Thus, the network is cost-effective since, for the same cost, significant indicators (including autonomy) showed an improvement. Nonetheless, the frequently cited hypothesis regarding differential transfers relative to spending was not confirmed. The planned evaluation of PRISMA France covers only the extent of network set-up, and no financial analysis is planned.

Fully integrated networks

An assessment of the transfer of resources between institutional and community care services by SIPA was carried out involving 1230 participants (Béland *et al.*, 2004, 2006). At each of the sites assessed, total costs were compared between a SIPA group and a control group, with the comparison limited to key services. The results are quite instructive since SIPA transfers an average sum of $7100 per patient from institutional services to local services, with total costs (including subsidies) exactly the same for the SIPA group and the control group and a health status that evolved in the same fashion for both the SIPA group and the control group. The money saved on residential care was $15 000 over 22 months for a single elderly person and $10 000 for an elderly person suffering from at least four chronic diseases. Furthermore, in the control group, there were twice as many people waiting for hospital beds, hospital stays were longer and hospitalisation costs were higher (increasing in proportion to the level of functional disability).

The On Lok programme evaluation (Yordi and Waldman, 1985) reveals positive results in terms of advantages for service users, a reduction in the rate of institutionalisation and a reduction in the total cost of around 21% per patient in the On Lok group. The estimated reduction in costs in the PACE programme was between 5 and 15% (Eng *et al.*, 1997). The results of the Social HMO project (version 1) were not positive in terms of hospitalisation or institutionalisation rates, and there was no reduction in the total cost of care (Kodner and Kyriacou, 2000). This has been explained (Johri *et al.*, 2003) by the absence of a genuinely multidisciplinary team. Moreover, the transfer expected between funding for the treatment of acute illness and funding for long-term care did not materialise because the case manager played more of an 'administrative' role, supporting geriatric care services rather than managing an integrated network. This function was more geared to setting up assessments and care plans to meet the needs of frail patients and checking the eligibility of participants in the network, without any real active involvement in coordinating integrated services or organising the provision of services. Under such conditions, the financial incentives inherent in the programme were ineffective. This relative failure led to a review of how Social HMOs were organised and the development of a second version of the Social HMO project. The main changes consist in improving the case manager's involvement, recalculating per capita payments on a basis more in line with the real risks and taking strong action in the area of primary care (training, assessment protocols, data gathering) to organise more proactive geriatric care with a view to reducing the need and the demand for treating acute cases and long-term care.

It has proved more difficult than expected to extend and develop the On Lok/PACE model and it has required expensive marketing drives (Branch *et al.*, 1995). In fact, inclusion in PACE networks has been limited, because the financial set-up for the project was good for people on low incomes relying on Medicare and Medicaid, whereas people on middle incomes had to make up a hefty difference (Bodenheimer, 1999). Also, patients' personal choices regarding GPs, specialists and nursing homes were very restricted. The Social HMO programme encountered similar problems. In the programmes funded by capitation, the determining factor is multiplication related to vulnerability that works to increase the contribution by the public health insurance fund (the Assurance Maladie in France or Medicare in the US) in funding the network. It also seems that not enough consideration has been given to the financial options and behaviour of patients who are not entitled to Medicaid.

The random assessment of the Rovereto experiment revealed excellent clinical and financial results (Bernabei *et al.*, 1998). Hospital admissions and placements in nursing homes were reduced and the cost per patient was $1800 lower compared with the control group (case managers' wages and coordination time were included in the cost analysis). The GPs' close involvement in the network and in-depth training for case managers apparently explains why the experiment was so successful (Bernabei *et al.*, 1998). The assessment of the Vittorio Veneto experiment (before and after assessment) also revealed positive results. Costs were cut by 29% (i.e. $1260 per patient) thanks to a reduction in the number and length of hospital stays. The development of an efficient system of home care reduced the number of inappropriate hospital stays for elderly patients, especially for those who, either for financial or social reasons, do not have access to primary care and for whom hospitals are the only option available in an emergency (Landi *et al.*, 1999).

Evaluating the networks

Evaluating these networks in cost-effectiveness terms is complex and there are a range of difficulties, of which the main appears to be providing a clear definition of the network's objectives. The network may in fact be focused on producing the range of services required for an easy transition from hospital to home, on organising an uninterrupted chain of services or on responding more directly to new demand (Leichsenring, 2007). The question of which indicators to use in this process is crucial. In practice, in current evaluations, the emphasis has been on how the network affects the health of the elderly and frail, hospitalisation rates, rates of institutionalisation in nursing homes and the differences in costs for patients treated

Table 8.1 Key themes from integrated health care networks.

The financial behaviour of the case manager	The different types of network are practically all based on the concept of case management. However, this role is not exactly the same in each model and is not always clearly specified. In some cases, the case manager is seen as fulfilling administrative tasks to determine whether patients are eligible and lightening the burden for health care providers. In other cases, it is his or her job to assign (assess and sort) patients to the various services. He or she may also help to strengthen network integration by bringing health care professionals together and coordinating the multidisciplinary team. He or she may also be responsible for controlling finances when called upon to deliver services to patients by contracting outside the network. The case manager may be appointed from among the health care professionals in the network, following further training. He or she may, on the other hand, come from outside, with a predominantly financial management background
The financial problem of inclusion	In practice, for the network to be financially viable, it must include enough service users to cover the network's fixed operating expenses thanks to money saved on treatment. Having a single point of access to the network makes inclusion much simpler since this solution has the merit of being visible. Standard assessment ensures that medical and social needs are targeted. Whether the patient can join the network or not depends on several factors: freedom of choice (particularly of GP) and choices made between the services available and the balance to be paid
The spread of networks	Whether an experimental network may become more widespread implies a need for precision and rigour in terms of financial results. Current results are generally short-term, which, to sum up, assess the transfer from the use of institutional services to local services. Various factors must be taken into consideration when looking toward long-term development: the pay-off of initial investments, the amount of time required for projects to become economically viable, the effects of financial incentives or pricing methods on the entire population, opinions on the fairness of the system and the differences in contributions made by frail people (Béland, 2007). The specific nature of the area in which experiments are developed further is also important. The cost of transport and, above all, non-use of services where physical and psychological distance is seen as too great may be obstacles to reproducing a successful experiment. More in-depth studies on the use of community care services with regard to distance and on the cost of distance or the economic geography of dependence are still needed
Capitation	The main difficulty in terms of this factor is the choice of levels. In the American networks, the capitation levels are calculated by referring to the cost of health care for a similar population group treated within the health system, using a factor of multiplication to take account of the specific nature of the network. Additional factors relate to two different levels: the choice of reference population group and in negotiating the multiplication factor
Resistance in the health care system	Flexibility of resources is one of the key elements in most of the networks studied. This introduces a form of market into the health care system, which presupposes that all stakeholders are not averse to playing a part in providing a fast response to satisfy demand and to transfer human and financial resources according to needs inside the health system network. If anyone in the health care system wishes to control his or her own budget and his or her own patients, the network will not be efficient. Resistance to change on the part of actors in the health care system should not be underestimated

within the network and those in a control group. Assessing the extent of network integration is a tricky task (Lombrail *et al.*, 2000; Fortanier *et al.*, 2005). In fact, the outcome of integrating different services must be defined, the levels and tasks involved in coordination must be described, levels of collaboration and confidence in the parties involved must be assessed – as must all the financial consequences. The more intensely integrated the network, the more necessary it is for the various stakeholders to agree on the assessment methods used (Leichsenring, 2007).

The issue of service users' financial participation is also vital. In the majority of evaluations, the only financial aspect analysed is public funding. The 'beneficiaries' of long-term care are seen as potentially financing their care, but not as economic actors able to make decisive financial choices. The financial behaviour of the users of these systems has not yet been studied in sufficient depth. The financial incentives imposed (pricing methods, access to care dependent on income, deductible amounts, liability for maintenance, drawing on the person's estate) affect the choices of care in ways that are not fully understood. There may be fundamental mismatches in understandings of health care (and its economic value) in the perceptions of service users and professionals, which may lead to contradictory behaviour between the beneficiaries of health care and health care providers. Insofar as methodology is concerned, it is extremely important that a good understanding of the advantages and added value for everyone involved in the complex process of co-production and co-consumption of long-term health care should be developed (Haverien and Tabibian, 2005). In the specifications for network objectives and assessment protocols, it is vital to include financial indicators relative to the advantages of each different category of participant.

From the evaluations outlined above, it appears that there are a range of key themes relating to finance which arise from integrated health care networks' (Table 8.1).

Conclusion

A range of different forms of networks for integrated care have emerged on a global scale, each of which has a range of different funding and structural challenges. Although the network is often presented as a form of ideal of economic perfection, this assumption is not necessarily borne out through the empirical literature. At the moment, there are a large range of networks whose economic impacts are difficult to evaluate due to insufficient data and because network targets are not sufficiently obvious. As a result, it remains difficult for governments to change the nature of their health care systems, to generalise successful experiences from individual integrated health care networks and to encourage medical teams to change their practice. Hardly surprisingly, therefore, many networks remain small and time limited, and it remains difficult to produce a definitive set of economic indicators which may facilitate quick and effective evaluation. To achieve this, networks will need to be seen not in isolation, but as part of wider social and political systems.

Summary

- There are different network funding models: public funding for good practice, funding coordinated health care programmes and funding totally integrated health care networks.
- The role of the case manager is not exactly the same in each model: to determine if patients are eligible, to assign patients to various services, to strength network integration, to control finances and so forth.
- Examples of public funding for good practice are gerontological networks in France, but there is no rigorous analysis assessing cost-effectiveness because of the lack of unified accounting follow-up.
- Coordinated care networks (such as the Darlington network, PRISMA and PRISMA France) improve significant indicators (including autonomy) and reduce hospitalisation rates for the same costs.
- Totally integrated health care networks may include a financial mechanism: such as capitation funding (e.g. On Lok, PACE, Social HMO and SIPA) or not (e.g. Rovereto and Vittorio Veneto networks).
- The integrated network is supposed to reduce recourse to emergency services and length of hospital stays and make more intensive use of local services. The per capita prepayment system is supposed to allow the transfer of resources from institutional services to local services.
- In the per capita system, the financial options and behaviour of patients who are not entitled to Medicaid are very important.
- Evaluating networks in cost-effectiveness terms requires a clear definition of the network's objectives.
- In current evaluations, the main indicators are the health of the elderly and frail, hospitalisation and institutionalisation in nursing homes rates, and the differences in costs for patients treated within the network and those in a control group.
- The financial behaviour of the users of networks (e.g. pricing methods and access to care dependent on income) affects the choice of care in ways that are not fully understood at present.

Further reading and resources

Useful sources on French networks include:

Daniel, C., Delpal, B. and Lannelongue, C. (2006) *Contrôle et evaluation du Fonds d'Aide à la Qualité des Soins de Ville (FAQSV) et de la Dotation de Développement des Réseaux (DDR)*. Paris, Rapport de Synthèse, Inspection Générale des Affaires Sociales.

DeStampa, M. *et al.* (2007) Modèle COPA-Ancrage (coordination, personnes âgées) coordination des services et gestion de cas, du modèle à l'évaluation. Paper presented at *International Symposium 'Réseaux de Santé, Intégration des Services Gérontologiques: Quel Modèle d'Evaluation?'* Paris, France, 21–22 June 2007.

Somme, D. *et al.* (2007) PRISMA France implanter c'est aussi innover! Présentation du programme d'implantation du modèle PRISMA de coordination dans le contexte français. Paper presented at *International Symposium 'Réseaux de Santé, Intégration des Services Gérontologiques: Quel Modèle d'Evaluation?'* Paris, France, 21–22 June 2007.

For a more general overview of some of the debates involved in the funding and delivery of primary health care, see:

Powell Davis, G. *et al.* (2006) *Coordination of Care within Primary Health Care and with Other Sectors: A Systematic Review.* Research Centre for Primary Health Care and Equity, School of Public Health and Community Medicine, University of New South Wales.

Relevant websites include:

SOLIDAGE is the website of the McGill University – Université de Montréal Research Group on Integrated Services for Older Persons, and is devoted to research, policy studies and practice development and training in the organisation, management and care of older people: http://www.solidage.ca. This website also contains extensive details on the SIPA project.

For more details on the PRISMA project, see http://www.usherbroke.ca/prisma or http://wwwprismaquebec.ca

The European Centre for Social Welfare Policy and Research provides expertise in the fields of welfare and social policy development – in particular in areas which call for multi- or interdisciplinary approaches, integrated policies and inter-sectoral action: http://www.euro.centre.org. This website also hosts the PROCARE research of Leichsenring and colleagues.

References

Béland, F. (2007) Comment évaluer les résultats des programmes en termes d'efficacité, de rendement, de performance. Paper presented at *International Symposium 'Réseaux de Santé, Intégration des Services Gérontologiques: Quel Modèle d'Evaluation?'*, Paris, France, 21–22 June 2007.

Béland, F. *et al.* (2004) *Évaluation du Système Intégré pour Personnes Agées Fragiles (SIPA): utilisation et coûts des services sociaux et de santé.* Montréal, Groupe de Recherche Université de Montréal-Université McGill sur les Services Intégrés pour les Personnes Agées.

Béland, F. *et al.* (2006) A system of integrated care for older persons with disabilities in Canada: results from a randomized controlled trial, *Journal of Gerontology: Medical Sciences*, 61(4), 367–373.

Bernabei, R. *et al.* (1998) Randomised trial of impact of model of integrated care and case management for older people living in the community, *British Medical Journal*, 316(7141), 1348–1351.

Bodenheimer, T. (1999) Long-term care for frail older people: the On Lok model, *New England Journal of Medicine*, 341, 1324–1328.

Branch, L. *et al.* (1995) The PACE evaluation: initial findings, *Gerontologist*, 35(3), 349–359.

Challis, D. *et al.* (1991) An evaluation of an alternative to long-stay hospital care for frail elderly patients. II Costs and effectiveness, *Age and Ageing*, 20(4), 245–254.

Challis, D. *et al.* (2006) Case management for older people: does integration make a difference? *Journal of Interprofessional Care*, 20(4), 335–348.

Daniel, C., Delpal, B. and Lannelongue, C. (2006) *Contrôle et evaluation du Fonds d'Aide à la Qualité des Soins de Ville (FAQSV) et de la Dotation de Développement des Réseaux (DDR)*. Paris, Rapport de Synthèse, Inspection Générale des Affaires Sociales.

DeStampa, M. *et al.* (2007) Modèle COPA-Ancrage (coordination, personnes âgées) coordination des services et gestion de cas, du modèle à l'évaluation. Paper presented at *International Symposium 'Réseaux de Santé, Intégration des Services Gérontologiques: Quel Modèle d'Evaluation?'* Paris, France, 21–22 June 2007.

Dominiak, A.L. *et al.* (2006) Evaluation économique des réseaux: apport d'expériences, *Journal d'Economie Médicale*, 24(7–8), 403–414.

Eng, C. *et al.* (1997) Program of all-inclusive care for the elderly (PACE): an innovative model of integrated geriatric care and financing, *Journal of the American Geriatrics Society*, 45(2), 223–232.

Esterman, A.J. and Ben-Tovim, D.I. (2002) The Australian coordinated care trials: success or failure? *Medical Journal of Australia*, 177, 469–470.

Fortanier, C. *et al.* (2005) Enjeux économiques des réseaux de santé: quelle evaluation? *Journal d'Economie Médicale*, 23(7–8), 415–424.

Haverin, R. and Tabibian, N. (2005) The outcomes and benefits of integrated care: in search of the service users' and carers' point of view, in J. Billings and K. Leichsenring (eds) *Integrating Health and Social Care Services for Older Persons: Evidence from Nine European Countries*. Aldershot, Ashgate.

Hébert, R. *et al.* (2003) PRISMA: a new model of integrated service delivery for the frail older people in Canada, *International Journal of Integrated Care*, 3. Available online via http://www.ijic.org

Johri, M., Béland, F. and Bergman, H. (2003) International experiments in integrated care for the elderly: a synthesis of evidence, *International Journal of Geriatric Psychiatry*, 18(3), 222–235.

Kane, R.L. *et al.* (1997) S/HMOs, the second generation: building on the experience of the first social health maintenance organisation demonstrations, *Journal of the American Geriatrics Society*, 45(1), 101–107.

Kodner, D.L. and Kyriacou, C.K. (2000) Fully integrated care for frail elderly: two American models, *International Journal of Integrated Care*, 1. Available online via http://www.ijic.org

Landi, F. *et al.* (1999) Impact of integrated home care services on hospital use, *Journal of the American Geriatrics Society*, 47(12), 1430–1434.

Lee, W. *et al.* (1998) PACE: a model for integrated care of frail older patients, *Geriatrics*, 53(6), 62–73.

Leichsenring, K. (2007) Les pistes différentes vers l'intégration des services sociaux et sanitaire en Europe: les résultats du projet PROCARE. Paper presented at *International Symposium 'Réseaux de Santé, Intégration des Services Gérontologiques: Quel Modèle d'Evaluation?'* Paris, France, 21–22 June 2007.

Leutz, W. (1999) Five laws for integrating medical and social services: lessons from the US and the UK, *Milbank Quaterly*, 77(1), 77–110.

Lombrail, P. *et al.* (2000) Benchmarks for evaluating health care networks, *Sante Publique*, 12(2), 161–176.

Somme, D. *et al.* (2007) PRISMA France implanter c'est aussi innover! Présentation du programme d'implantation du modèle PRISMA de coordination dans le contexte français. Paper presented at *International Symposium 'Réseaux de Santé, Intégration des Services Gérontologiques: Quel Modèle d'Evaluation ?'* Paris, France, 21–22 June 2007.

Yordi, C.L. and Waldman, J. (1985) A consolidated model of long-term care: service utilization and cost impacts, *The Gerontologist*, 25(4), 389–397.

9 Self-management with others: the role of partnerships in supporting self-management for people with long-term conditions

Gawaine Powell Davies, Sarah Dennis and Christine Walker

Box 9.1   Why self-management matters.

I had a heart attack in 1994 and did a 6-week rehab course at a local hospital and then I fended for myself for the next 8 years. At the end of 2001 I had another heart attack and then pulmonary oedema. I was told it was chronic heart failure and I thought that the was it, I'd die. It transpired that the second heart attack was the best thing that happened to me because the treating hospital referred me to the community health service for an exercise program. I had to wait a few months before I could get in (I got annoyed about it at the time and complained) but I started off in a supervised group. That was about 3 or 4 years ago and then we decided to break free and become a self-managed group. Some people felt consternation because they lost their 'security blanket' of the supervision but regardless of that we have advanced to two groups a week. I have just come from the Friday group. We have exercises but we also have social activities. The eldest member is 84 and the youngest 52. If someone doesn't attend, then a member of the group contacts them to see they are OK. The groups are also part of Heart Support Australia and that's further support. As an individual, the best thing that happened to me was the referral to an exercise program and being able to form a self-management group. The community health service gave us the front door key so we start at 7.30 am with warm up exercises and at the end of the morning we all go for a long walk together. I no longer smoke or drink, the group is now the focus of my life. I now get on with my life.

Man aged 71 in Victoria, Australia, speaking about his view of self-management, November 2006 (Chronic Illness Alliance, 2006).

Good self-management is an important part of the treatment of long-term conditions. It is one of the processes through which people come to terms with their condition and its impact on their lives. It can contribute to improved health outcomes through greater adherence to evidence-based care (Weingarten *et al.*, 2002) and help reduce risk by tackling the behavioural risk factors that contribute to chronic disease, particularly in developed countries (Lorig *et al.*, 1999a). A focus on self-management also fits with prevailing social attitudes: that health care should be consumer-focused, and that people have significant responsibility for maintaining their own health.

As the story at the start of this chapter reminds us (see Box 9.1), people do not manage their long-term conditions alone, but in social contexts and with the support of health care providers. After his first heart attack, the man felt helpless when he was 'left to fend for himself'. Following his second heart attack, he was introduced to the primary health care system, with its secondary prevention and self-management programmes, and through this to a group of others with chronic conditions. They began an exercise programme under the supervision of a health professional, but as their confidence grew, they decided to 'break free' and run it themselves, under the umbrella of Heart Support Australia. Together they created a social partnership in which the man was both a receiver and a giver of support. At the end of the story he no longer smokes or drinks, but this appears to be secondary to the sense of solidarity and control that the group has given him: 'I now get on with my life'. This man's experience gives a vivid picture of how important partnerships with service providers and with others with the condition can be to sustaining self-management over the long-term.

In this chapter the authors will explore the components of self-management and the role of partnerships in supporting these. This will be related to chronic disease management policies in the UK, the US, New Zealand, the Netherlands and Australia. In many ways, the scope of the partnerships to support self-management discussed here is broader than those discussed in some other chapters, focusing on relationships between services and service users, rather than solely on relationships between different services.

Definition of self-management and related concepts

At the core of the concept of self-management is the notion of a person taking active steps to manage an aspect of their health and taking responsibility for their daily care needs (Walker, 2003). This involves learning the skills and gaining the confidence to manage the condition and to live with it as part of their life. Gruman and Von Korff (1996) define self-management as:

> Engaging in activities that protect and promote health, monitoring and managing of symptoms and signs of illness, managing the impacts of illness on functioning, emotions, interpersonal relationships and adhering to regimes.

Self-management must address the person's condition and its treatment, fit with their lifestyle and social circumstances and take account of the health care that they are receiving. It may be needed to manage an existing condition or to prevent the onset of disease and involve issues that are specific to that condition or apply more generally to living with a chronic illness (Wagner and Groves, 2002). The condition may impact on the person's family or the wider community, and these may have a role to play in supporting self-management. *Self-management support* is the assistance that people with long-term conditions receive from health professionals and others, including family members, friends and the community, to assist them to better manage their health (Von Korff *et al.*, 1997). Those providing assistance may themselves need support: for example, teachers may need training in how to help children with asthma manage their condition at school. Self-management support may include providing information about the specific medical condition and its treatment, giving broader education to build health literacy, developing the skills the person needs to monitor and manage their condition and providing support and encouragement. It can be seen as an adaptation of the normal role of a health professional to the requirements of chronic disease care.

The role of self-management in chronic disease care

In developed countries, there has been a marked shift in chronic disease care from a reactive system with a focus on acute care to one that is structured, proactive and designed to support the management of conditions over a long period of time. The Chronic Care Model developed by Wagner and colleagues (1996) describes the essential elements, including self-management support and an organised health care system. The Expanded Chronic Care Model extends this to include population health approaches (Barr *et al.*, 2003). This model makes the role of partnerships and networks in self-management support explicit (Figure 9.1). At the core of the model is the person with chronic condition, supported by an activated community, and the practice team, supported by partner organisations. Self-management support comes from within the health care system and through supportive policies, environments and action within the community. This is broadly consistent with the World Health Organisation's (2002) Innovative Care for Chronic Conditions model, which describes a triad of care between the individual and their family, the community in which they live and the health care system.

A recent systematic review of chronic disease management using the Chronic Care Model as a framework for analysis found that self-management support was the most common component of effective chronic disease management programmes (Zwar *et al.*, 2006; Dennis *et al.*, 2008). The impact was not consistent across all conditions and favoured strategies for developing self-efficacy for specific elements of self-management, such as exercise or diet.

Supporting self-management: the role of partnerships and networks

The Expanded Chronic Care Model highlights three areas for partnerships and associated networks: between the person with a chronic condition and their health

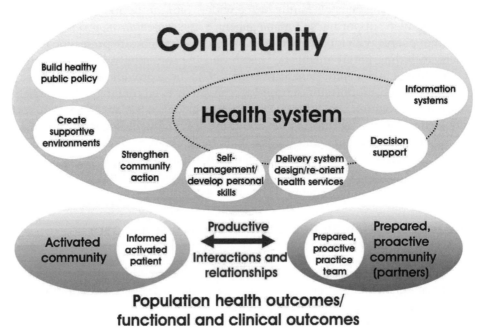

Figure 9.1   The Expanded Chronic Care Model. (Source: Barr *et al.*, 2003; reproduced with permission.)

care providers; the communities and social networks to which they belong; and between the person's immediate health care providers and other health and community organisations. This section reviews each of these in turn.

People with chronic conditions and their health care providers

Self-management is usually supported through the person's health care providers (Harvey and Docherty, 2007) or leaders of self-management programmes such as the UK's Expert Patient Programme (Department of Health, 2001). The relationship will vary according to the characteristics and expectations of the people involved: for example, self-management support may be less effective if differences in cultural or linguistic background are not taken into account (Office for Aboriginal and Torres Strait Islander Health, 2001). Bodenheimer *et al.* (2002a) characterise the relationship needed to support self-management as a partnership where the provider recognises the person as an expert on their own condition. It is ultimately the person who sets the goals, and the provider assists them to achieve these through education and support (Battersby and the SA HealthPlus Team, 2005) and shared decision-making (Montori *et al.*, 2006). Unlike traditional patient education, the focus is on teaching problem-solving skills and building self-efficacy rather than simply providing information and developing technical skills (Bodenheimer *et al.*, 2002a).

This is a joint activity requiring a degree of continuity of care, which may be strengthened by using systematic follow-up and reminders. This provides regular opportunities to review a self-care regime or to build up to a lifestyle change such as stopping smoking. Continuity may be with a single provider, but where a person is receiving care from multiple (and often diverse) providers, the emphasis is on consistency of information and teamwork to ensure continuity across boundaries (Freeman *et al.*, 2003). This can be facilitated by working to common standards and using consistent education materials. Although having a variety of service providers may make continuity harder to achieve, it may also provide an opportunity to seek different elements of support from the sources where the person feels most comfortable.

People with chronic conditions in their social settings

People self-manage their chronic conditions in normal social contexts and as part of their daily life. The potential for supportive partnerships and networks extends across all the settings where the impact of a chronic condition is felt (Segal, 2007). The following sections illustrate this in relation to the family; workplace, school and social partnerships; the broader community; and self-help networks.

The family

Families and other close relationships play an important overall role in supporting health. For men, being married is in itself protective for good general health (Lilliard and Waite, 1995); older women are more likely to live alone and to require outside care when they fall ill or become frail (Broom, 1998). In studies from the US, patients with heart disease who did not have a spouse or other significant relationship were less likely to survive for 5 years following an event than those who did (Williams *et al.*, 1992). The family is likely to be the arena for much self-management and a source of self-management support. Self-monitoring and treatment regimes may become part of the family routine, and changes to patterns of diet and exercise may need the support of the family as a whole. A review article on psycho-social barriers to diabetes self-management (Glasgow *et al.*, 2001) found that low levels of family social support acted as a barrier to effective self-management. An Australian project to evaluate self-management support for indigenous Australians found that many had a dysfunctional family life which had a negative impact on their ability to manage their chronic disease (Collins, 2003).

It is interesting to note that while Duckett (2000) and others have emphasised the role of the family in health outcomes, self-management programmes such as the Expert Patient Programme (Department of Health) and the Chronic Disease Self-Management Program (Lorig *et al.*, 2001) continue to work with the person with the chronic condition in isolation. Where partnerships are discussed directly, these tend to relate to partnerships with health professionals in the community rather than to partnerships with family members (Harvey and Docherty, 2007).

Workplace, school and social partnerships

The extent to which people with long-term conditions involve their workplace, school and social partnerships will depend in part on the specific details of their condition and how they wish to manage it. The role of schools and workplaces has been explored in the context of diabetes self-management (Norris *et al.*, 2002). In the workplace setting, self-management education involving co-workers was found to increase their tolerance to the difficulties of having diabetes and led to improved productivity by the person with diabetes. However, this was accompanied by issues concerning confidentiality and labelling that need to be taken into account. Similar results and barriers were identified with school support for diabetes self-management. In an environment such as a children's camp, there is evidence that self-management support improves the knowledge of children with diabetes or asthma and provides an opportunity for them to explore how controlling their disease can fit safely around exciting activities.

There have also been school-based programmes to support asthma self-management in Australia which have demonstrated improved quality of life and reduced school absenteeism in those attending the programme (Shah *et al.*, 2001). The Asthma Friendly Schools Programme has been funded by the Australian Government Department of Health and Ageing since 2000, and by 2007 more than half of all schools had received training and were asthma friendly. Self-management support fits well within the concept of the health-promoting school, which builds health promotion into the formal and informal curriculum in the school, the school ethos and its relationship with the community.

The broader community

The Expanded Chronic Care Model highlights the scope for community-level action to support self-management through healthy public policy. This may involve programmes for people with chronic conditions such as exercise classes, indirectly through provision of healthy environments such as smoke-free zones or safe places to walk. Community action may be facilitated where there is a defined community to which the person relates. For example, a number of remote indigenous communities in Australia with high rates of diabetes have succeeded in improving diabetes control by ensuring that healthy food is available at a reasonable price through the community general store (Rowley *et al.*, 2000). Self-management support from within the community has been shown to be effective for groups who may otherwise be difficult to reach and those who are culturally and linguistically diverse, where information can be provided in the community language and in a culturally appropriately manner. Pre-existing programmes can be adapted to work effectively in specific programmes: for example, the Stanford Chronic Disease Self-Management Program has been revised for Hispanic (Lorig *et al.*, 1999b) and Vietnamese communities in the US and has been extensively revised and run in Shanghai (Dongbo *et al.*, 2003).

Although these programmes report similar results to other self-management programmes delivered in English, there are still gaps in our understanding of how well programmes work across diverse ethnic communities (Walker, 2003). A peer-led Self-Management of Chronic Illness project was carried out in the Chinese, Vietnamese, Italian and Greek populations of Melbourne, Australia. The programme was successful in attracting participants and improving general health and self-efficacy, but found cultural differences in what participants most valued: Chinese and Vietnamese people responded to the emphasis on physical exercise, while Greek and Italian people were more concerned about social isolation (Swerissen et al., 2006). A peer-led self-management programme for Bangladeshis in the UK was also reported as successful (Griffiths et al., 2005). However it was not integrated into the rest of the health care system, and as a result had a high drop-out rate and no reduction in health service use. These two pieces of research suggest that self-management programmes need to be relevant to the community and integrated into the primary health care system particularly if they aim to reach the more marginal groups in our communities.

Self-help networks

In the story at the beginning of this chapter (see Box 9.1), the exercise group changed over time from a professional-led group to a self-help group. Self-help, self-care or mutual help groups have been defined as groups of peers who utilise their experiences to support and advise others whilst receiving support and advice themselves (Woolacott et al., 2006). They provide structures through which people who have the same chronic condition can support each other in living with their condition. The self-help movement is large and diverse with groups for almost every medical condition.

The evidence for the effectiveness of self-help groups is mixed: US research into support groups for people with mental health conditions has demonstrated that those who attended the groups had fewer hospitalisations, shorter hospital stays and less contact with the mental health system than those who did not (Edmundson et al., 1982). In Australia, membership of the support group GROW was associated with improved well-being and a sense of self as well as reduced hospitalisations (Finn et al., 2007). However, a recent review of the literature found few well-designed studies of self-care support networks and therefore weak evidence for their effectiveness (Woolacott et al., 2006). Arguably these methodological issues are typical of the partnership field more generally (see chapter 11 for further details on these issues.)

The self-help movement makes extensive use of the internet, something which is not always comfortable for service providers (see Box 9.2).

In 2004 some 25 000 health and wellness support groups were listed on Yahoo! Groups and many people have benefited from online support (Eysenbach et al., 2004). Ferguson noted that partnerships between medical practitioners and online support groups could be beneficial too (Ferguson, 2000). Consumers could access support and information for which medical practitioners did not have the time, and medical practitioners could help ensure the quality of online information. In 2004 he reported that 'e-patients' were using the internet for information and relying on online support groups for emotional support, referrals to specialists

> **Box 9.2**   Use of the internet.
>
> I knew that many patients with chronic diseases had been making use of online medi-
> cal information. Nonetheless, I was shocked, fascinated, and more than a bit confused
> by what I saw. I'd been trained in the old medical school style: my instructors had
> insisted that patients could not be trusted to understand or manage complex medical
> matters. Thinking back through my years of training and practice, I realized that there
> had always been an unspoken prohibition against groups of patients getting together.
> I had the uncomfortable sense that by promoting interactions between patients and
> de-emphasizing the central role of the physician, I might be violating some deep taboo.
> (Hoch and Ferguson, 2005)

and medical advice (Ferguson and Frydmann, 2004). For further discussion of
partnership working and IT, see Chapter 7.

Networks for service providers

The Expanded Chronic Care Model showed the 'prepared proactive practice team'
as part of a larger network. This can include not only the 'community partners'
noted in the diagram but also other service providers and support organisations.
This larger network may have a number of purposes. One is to provide support
to the health care provider in the form of training, advice or support: for example, in Australia, Diabetes Australia trains practice nurses as diabetes educators
and the Heart Foundation provides education materials and brief intervention
programmes for a health care provider to use. The network can also provide information about access to referral services such as education programmes and self-
help groups, and ethnic-specific organisations that may support self-management
within their own communities.

Partnerships between service providers can help ensure that the person with
a long-term chronic condition receives consistent information and advice. Conflicting information may be confusing and undermine the person's efforts at self-
management. There is an important role for organisations such as the National Institute of Health and Clinical Excellence (NIHCE) in the UK and the National Institute
for Clinical Studies (NICS) in Australia to identify and promulgate evidence-based
approaches to management and self-management.

Policy supporting self-management partnerships

Many countries have recognised the importance of self-management and instituted
policies and programmes to encourage its development. While a number have
focused on establishing discrete self-management education programmes such as
the Lorig programme, some have also focused on the partnerships and networks
needed to support self-management. This section provides a brief summary of some

international programmes and policies for supporting partnerships and networks for self-management.

Australia

The Australian health system is a complex mixture of state and federal responsibilities with both public and private providers. Both the state and federal governments support self-management as an integral part of chronic disease management but do not endorse a single model, leading to a variety of different approaches.

The Sharing Health Care Initiative (1999–2007) funded 12 demonstration projects of chronic disease self-management, addressing a range of chronic conditions. Projects have included education and training for both patients and health professionals, developing social networks for people with long-term conditions and referral networks. Self-management education programmes have used both the Stamford Model (Lorig et al., 1999a) and the Flinders Model (Battersby and the SA HealthPlus Team, 2005), both of which involve partnerships and goal setting.

A number of initiatives in recent years have supported more coordinated chronic disease care and facilitated partnerships between service providers. The Enhanced Primary Care package supports general practitioners (GPs) to develop collaborative multidisciplinary care plans with other service providers, and funding is available to support access to allied health care. The Australian Better Health Initiative, a 5-year package aimed at reducing the impact of chronic disease, includes support for lifestyle change through individual and group lifestyle education and training for health professionals (including GPs) in teaching self-management skills.

The UK

The UK has chosen to support partnerships between people with chronic disease through the Expert Patient Programme (Department of Health, 2001), developed following the influential work of the Long-Term Medical Conditions Alliance. This is a 6-week generic training programme where people with a chronic disease are trained to deliver self-management education and support to other adults with chronic conditions. It has been run widely in Primary Care Trust sites but does not directly involve a partnership with the GP. A recent evaluation showed improvements in self-efficacy and energy, and fewer social role limitations, better psychological well being, more exercise, relaxation and greater participation with clinicians, but no significant difference in use of health services (Kennedy et al., 2007).

New Zealand

Partnerships have been a key feature of policy and programmes in New Zealand, particularly for engaging people from disadvantaged backgrounds with health professionals. In 2004 the New Zealand Ministry of Health launched Care Plus, a new service for people with chronic disease delivered through primary health organisations (Ministry of Health, 2004). The key feature of the Care Plus programme was identifying people with chronic disease who required intensive case management. GPs who served a population with a higher proportion of Pacific Islander, Maori or low socio-economic status were able to receive additional capitation funding to support care (McAvoy and Coster, 2005). Other partnerships between the primary health organisations and local health authority have been established locally with the aim of providing the 'seamless' delivery of health care for people with chronic diseases, particularly those from disadvantaged communities such as the Counties Manukau region in South Auckland (Wellingham *et al.*, 2003).

The US

The fragmented nature of the US health care system makes it difficult to introduce policy to support self-management on a broad scale. However, many of the managed care organisations have included self-management support as part of implementing the Chronic Care Model for people with chronic conditions (Bodenheimer *et al.*, 2002b). Many of the initiatives with a large self-management component have targeted groups such as African Americans or Hispanic populations who frequently live below the poverty line and do not have access to health insurance.

The Netherlands

Partnerships have been an important feature of chronic disease management in the Netherlands. Transmural care was developed in the 1990s to address the gap between hospital and primary care and the separate funding systems (van der Linden *et al.*, 2001). Nurses, some with specialist training, play an important role in many of the programmes, working in partnership with people with chronic disease to provide education and family support. Some regions have combined the transmural model with disease management: for example, disease management has been developed for diabetes in the Maastricht region (Vrijhoef *et al.*, 2001). This grew out of an earlier shared care model involving specialist nurses and hospital specialists, which has been extended to include a broader team of health care professionals (GP, practice nurse, specialist nurse and endocrinologist). The involvement of care providers depends on the severity of the patient's condition, with greater emphasis on hospital-led care for those with more severe conditions.

Critique, future options and developments

The chapter began with the experience of a man coming to terms with his heart condition, supported by health professionals and a self-help group. This led into a discussion of the Expanded Chronic Care Model, which highlights the value of partnerships involving people with chronic conditions, their primary health professional, their family and broader social networks to support self-management. The model emphasises the need for a supportive network for health professionals. It also recognises the role of the broader social context and wider community: they may be supportive to the person with a long-term condition, or indifferent or even hostile, particularly when there is stigma attached to the condition as with HIV/ AIDS or mental illness.

Self-management is important, but should be seen in context. Self-management support is only one part of the care that people need for chronic conditions, and it does not take the place of high-quality medical treatment. People vary in their capacity for self-management, and not everyone will be able to manage their condition effectively. Self-management support should therefore not be treated as a substitute for professional care, nor should it be used to transfer costs from one part of the health system to another or to shift the burden from service providers to consumers. It is an adjunct to professional health care and not a substitute for it.

There is much that we do not yet understand about self-management and about the partnerships needed to support this way of working. Whilst there has been considerable research into discrete self-management programmes for specific conditions, there has been less research into the role of families, workplaces and self-help groups to support self-management. Little is known about how best to develop and sustain partnerships, particularly through community organisations, and how these can be used to provide sustainable infrastructure for self-management support. We need to understand better how to design programmes to meet the needs of socially and ethnically diverse communities, especially for indigenous and non-English-speaking communities, many with high rates of chronic disease, and how to engage their particular social networks in self-management support.

Self-management support reflects many of the challenges posed by chronic disease. Health systems have to take on unfamiliar roles and develop partnerships with organisations outside normal health service networks. People with a chronic condition may need to look for support in settings with no existing role in health care. Community networks and organisations may need to learn about chronic conditions and find ways of supporting their members, but the partnerships thus formed will be an important part of the response to an increasing burden of chronic disease.

Summary

- Self-management support is becoming an important component in the management of chronic disease in developed countries.
- Self-care strategies may improve when people with chronic illnesses have access to a variety of self-management supports.
- Self-management support and support programmes have positive outcomes in terms of increased self-efficacy and better health care management in a variety of chronic conditions, but there is little evidence of impact on service utilisation.
- Self-management requires support from the family and the wider community in addition to support from health professionals.
- Peer-led self-management programmes and support groups are effective means of improving individuals' self-management.

- The internet is used widely for self-management programmes, including chat groups and formal self-management programmes, and may be particularly valuable for those who are isolated.
- More research is needed to understand the impact of partnerships on the ability of the person to self-manage their condition and on supporting self-management in culturally and linguistically diverse communities.

Further reading and useful websites

Useful sources include:

Barr, V.J. *et al.* (2003) The expanded chronic care model: an integration of concepts and strategies from population health promotion and chronic care model, *Hospital Quarterly*, 7, 73–82.

Bodenheimer, T. *et al.* (2002) Patient self-management of chronic disease in primary care, *Journal of the American Medical Association*, 288, 2469–2475.

Norris, S.L. *et al.* (2002) Increasing diabetes self-management education in community settings: a systematic review, *American Journal of Preventive Medicine*, 22, 39–66.

Wagner, E.H. and Groves, T. (2002) Care for chronic diseases, *British Medical Journal*, 325, 913–914.

Walker, C. *et al.* (2003) *Chronic Illness: New Perspectives, New Directions*. Melbourne, Tertiary Press.

Walker, C., Swerissen, H. and Belfrage, J. (2003) Self-management: its place in the management of chronic illnesses, *Australian Health Review*, 26, 34–42.

Weingarten, S. R. *et al.* (2002) Interventions used in disease management programmes for patients with chronic illness – which ones work? Meta-analysis of published reports, *British Medical Journal*, 325, 925–933.

Zwar, N. *et al.* (2006) *A Systematic Review of Chronic Disease Management*. Research Centre for Primary Health Care and Equity, School of Public Health and Community Medicine, University of New South Wales. Available online via http://www.anu.edu.au/aphcri/Domain/ChronicDiseaseMgmt/Approved_25_Zwar.pdf

Relevant websites include:

British Columbia's Chronic Disease Management Program (especially for the Expanded Chronic Care Model): http://www.health.gov.bc.ca/cdm/cdminbc/chronic_care_model.html

Chronic Illness Alliance: http://www.chronicillness.org.au (see also the Special Interest Group at http://www.chronicillness.org.au/sig)

Flinders Human Behaviour and Health Research Unit: http://som.flinders.edu.au/FUSA/CCTU/

(Australian Government) Health Insite website: http://www.healthinsite.gov.au/

(US) Improving Chronic Illness Care: http://www.improvingchroniccare.org/

Institute for Healthcare Improvement: http://www.ihi.org/IHI/Topics/PatientCentered-Care/SelfManagementSupport/

Interdisciplinary Research Centre in Health at Coventry University: http://www.corporate.coventry.ac.uk/cms/jsp/polopoly.jsp?d=796&a=11575

International Disease Management Alliance: http://www.dmalliance.org

Long-term Conditions Alliance: http://www.lmca.org.uk/

National Primary Care Research and Development Centre at Manchester University: http://
www.npcrdc.ac.uk

Stamford University Patient Education Centre: http://patienteducation.stanford.edu/
index.html

References

Barr, V.J. *et al.* (2003) The expanded chronic care model: an integration of concepts and strategies from population health promotion and chronic care model, *Hospital Quarterly*, 7, 73–82.

Battersby, M.W. and The SA HealthPlus Team (2005) Health reform through coordinated care: SA HealthPlus, *British Medical Journal*, 330, 662–665.

Bodenheimer, T., Lorig, K., Holman, H. and Grumbach, K. (2002a) Patient self-management of chronic disease in primary care, *Journal of the American Medical Association*, 288, 2469–2475.

Bodenheimer, T., Wagner, E.H. and Grumbach, K. (2002b) Improving primary care for patients with chronic illness, *Journal of the American Medical Association*, 288, 1775–1779.

Broom, D. (1998) Facing facts, facing futures: challenges to women's health, *Journal of Primary Health Interchange*, 4, 40–49.

Chronic Illness Alliance (2006) *Transcript of Focus Group on Behalf of Knox Community Health Service*. Victoria, Australia, Chronic Illness Alliance.

Collins, J. (2003) *Eyre Peninsula Chronic Disease Self-Management Project for Aboriginal Communities in Ceduna/Koonibba and Port Lincoln*. Report to South Australian Department of Human Services. South Australia, Eyre Peninsula Division of General Practice.

Dennis, S., Zwar, N., Griffiths, R., Roland, M., Hasan, I., Powell Davies, G. (2008) Chronic disease management in primary care: from evidence to policy, MJA, 188 (8 suppl) 553–556.

Department of Health (2001) *The Expert Patient: A New Approach to Chronic Disease Management for the 21st Century*. London, Department of Health.

Dongbo, F. *et al.* (2003) Implementation and quantitative evaluation of a chronic disease self-management programme in Shanghai, China: a randomized controlled trial, *Bulletin of World Health Organization*, 81, 174–182.

Duckett, S. (2000) *The Australian Health Care System*. Oxford, Oxford University Press.

Edmundson, E. *et al.* (1982) Integrating skill building and peer supporting mental health treatment: the early intervention and community development projects, in M. Jeger and R. Slotnick (eds) *Community Mental Health and Behavioral Ecology*. New York, Plenum Press.

Eysenbach, G. *et al.* (2004) Health related virtual communities and electronic support groups: systematic review of on-line peer to peer interactions, *British Medical Journal*, 328, 1166–1170.

Ferguson, T. (2000) On-line patient-helpers and physicians working together: a new partnership for high quality care, *British Medical Journal*, 321, 1129–1132.

Ferguson, T. and Frydmann, G. (2004) The first generation of e-patients, *British Medical Journal*, 328, 1148–1149.

Finn, L., Bishop, B. and Sparrow, N.H. (2007) Mutual help groups: an important gateway to wellbeing and mental health, *Australian Health Review*, 31, 246–255.

Freeman, G., Oleson, F. and Hjortdahl, P. (2003) Continuity of care: an essential element in modern general practice, *Family Practice*, 20, 623–627.

Glasgow, R.E., Toobert, D.J. and Gillette, C.D. (2001) Psychosocial barriers to diabetes self-management and quality of life, *Diabetes Spectrum*, 14, 33–41.

Griffiths, C. *et al.* (2005) Randomised controlled trial of a lay-led self-management programme for Bangladeshi patients with chronic disease, *British Journal of General Practice*, 55, 831–837.

Gruman, J. and Von Korff, M. (1996) *Indexed Bibliography on Self-Management for People with Chronic Diseases*. Washington DC, Center for Advancement in Health.

Harvey, P. and Docherty, B. (2007) Sysiphus and self-management: the chronic condition self-management paradox, *Australian Health Review*, 31, 184–192.

Hoch, D. and Ferguson, T. (2005) What I've learned from e-patients, *PLoS Medicine*, 2, e206.

Kennedy, A. *et al.* (2007) The effectiveness and cost effectiveness of a national lay-led self care support programme for patients with long term conditions: a pragmatic randomized controlled trial, *Journal of Epidemiology and Community Health*, 61, 254–261.

Lilliard, L. and Waite, L. (1995) Til death do us part: marital disruption and mortality, *American Journal of Sociology*, 100, 1131–1156.

Lorig, K. *et al.* (1999a) Evidence suggesting that a chronic disease self-management program can improve health status while reducing hospitalization: a randomized trial, *Medical Care*, 37, 5–14.

Lorig, K. *et al.* (2001) Chronic disease self-management program: two-year health status and health care utilization outcomes, *Medical Care*, 39, 1217–1223.

Lorig, K., Gonzalez, V. and Ritter, P. (1999b) Community-based Spanish language arthritis education program: a randomized trial, *Medical Care*, 37, 957–963.

Mcavoy, B. and Coster, G. (2005) General practice and the New Zealand health reforms – lessons for Australia? *Australia and New Zealand Health Policy*, 2, 26.

Ministry of Health (2004) *Care Plus: An Overview*. Wellington, New Zealand, Ministry of Health.

Montori, V., Gafni, A. and Charles, C. (2006) A shared treatment decision-making approach between patients with chronic conditions and their clinicians: the case of diabetes, *Health Expectations*, 9, 25–36.

Norris, S.L. *et al.* (2002) Increasing diabetes self-management education in community settings: a systematic review, *American Journal of Preventive Medicine*, 22, 39–66.

Office for Aboriginal and Torres Strait Islander Health (2001) *Better Health Care: Studies in the Successful Delivery of Primary Health Care Services for Aboriginal and Torres Strait Islander Australians*. Canberra, Commonwealth Department of Health and Aged Care.

Rowley, K. *et al.* (2000) Effectiveness of a community-directed 'healthy lifestyle' program in a remote Australian aboriginal community, *Australian and New Zealand Journal of Public Health*, 24, 136–144.

Segal, J. (2007) 'Compliance' to 'Concordance': a critical view, *Journal of Medical Humanities*, 28, 81–96.

Shah, S. *et al.* (2001) Effect of peer led program for asthma education in adolescents: cluster randomised control trial, *British Medical Journal*, 322(7286), 583–585.

Swerissen, H. *et al.* (2006) A randomised control trial of a self-management program for people with a chronic illness from Vietnamese, Chinese, Italian and Greek backgrounds, *Patient Education and Counselling*, 64, 360–368.

van Der Linden, B.A., Spreeuwenberg, C. and Schrijvers, A.J.P. (2001) Integration of care in the Netherlands: the development of transmural care since 1994, *Health Policy*, 55, 111–120.

Von Korff, M. *et al.* (1997) Collaborative management of chronic illness, *Annals of Internal Medicine*, 127, 1097–1102.

Vrijhoef, H.J.M. *et al.* (2001) Adoption of disease management model for diabetes in region of Maastricht, *British Medical Journal*, 323, 983–985.

Wagner, E., Austin, B. and Von Korff, M. (1996) Organizing care for patients with chronic illness, *Milbank Quarterly*, 74, 511–544.

Wagner, E.H. and Groves, T. (2002) Care for chronic diseases, *British Medical Journal*, 325, 913–914.

Walker, C. (2003) Putting 'self' back into self-management, in C. Walker (ed.) *Chronic Illness: New Perspectives and New Directions*. Victoria, Australia Tertiary Press.

Weingarten, S.R. *et al.* (2002) Interventions used in disease management programmes for patients with chronic illness – which ones work? Meta-analysis of published reports, *British Medical Journal*, 325, 925–933.

Wellingham, J. *et al.* (2003) The development and implementation of the Chronic Care Management Programme in Counties Manukau, *New Zealand Medical Journal*, 116, U327.

Williams, R. *et al.* (1992) Prognostic importance of social and economic resources among medically treated patients with angiographically documented coronary heart disease, *Journal of the American Medical Association*, 267, 520–524.

Woolacott, N. *et al.* (2006) *Systematic Review of the Clinical Effectiveness of Self Care Support Networks in Health and Social Care*. York, Centre for Reviews and Dissemination.

World Health Organisation (2002) *Innovative Care for Chronic Conditions: Building Blocks for Action – Global Report*. Geneva, World Health Organisation.

Zwar, N. *et al.* (2006) *A Systematic Review of Chronic Disease Management*. Research Centre for Primary Health Care and Equity, School of Public Health and Community Medicine, University of New South Wales. Available online via http://www.anu.edu.au/aphcri/Domain/ChronicDiseaseMgmt/Approved_25_Zwar.pdf

10 Self-directed support as a framework for partnership working

John O'Brien and Simon Duffy

While several other chapters in this book explore 'partnership working' from the perspective of the health and social care system, we approach this issue from the perspective of the citizen. In particular, we focus on those citizens who have significant impairments and need significant levels of support in order to achieve independent living. We will argue that from this perspective, the goal of achieving system integration between different agencies (e.g. between health and social care systems) can seem either redundant or unhelpful. Instead, what seems to matter more is a personalised integration of supports that can only be achieved with the active participation of the citizen (Duffy, 2004). The ability to achieve personalised integration is a function of systems that put power and control in the hands of the citizen, enable full access to the widest range of services and opportunities and develop the communities that can take advantage of these opportunities. Although these issues are common in many developed countries, our focus here is mainly on the UK and the US (since these countries both have a relatively long history of piloting and, to some extent, evaluating new initiatives in this area).

On this understanding, current efforts to promote the system integration of service delivery agencies may even be an obstacle to genuine progress, locking people into a narrower range of options (see Figure 10.1). If this understanding is correct then the energy that has been focused on system integration could instead shift to moving the whole service system to operate and respond to self-directed supports, thus enabling citizens who require personal assistance to be in control of their own lives and to assume a share of responsibility for achieving personalised integration.

In this framework, partnership efforts must become sufficiently courageous and competent to accomplish three difficult things:

- Guide themselves by adopting the way of thinking exemplified by the British government in *Improving the Life Chances of Disabled People* (Cabinet Office, 2005). This document focuses not on ill health or individual impairment, but on the social and political changes needed to ensure that disabled citizens have the same 'life chances' as non-disabled people. This will enable the hard work of

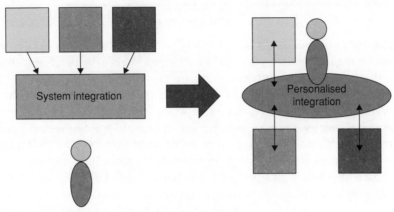

Figure 10.1   From system to personalised integration.

uprooting policies and practices based on the presumption that need for assistance diminishes the responsibilities and rights of citizenship. It also allows rethinking historical distinctions between health and social care in a way that more clearly distinguishes treatment for ill health from support for everyday life.
- Embrace the spirit of the UK Disability Discrimination Act (which prohibits discrimination against disabled people). All services that wish to comply will learn how to capably perform their particular tasks in a way that is accessible to all people with impairments. In the long term, this is an even more important outcome than collaboration among service agencies.
- Mobilise people who commission social care, people who manage and offer social care, and people who rely on social care to learn the ways of thinking, roles and practices necessary to realise fully the benefits of the strategic direction set in the UK policy documents *Improving the Life Chances of Disabled People* and *Our Health, Our Care, Our Say* (Department of Health, 2006) (Box 10.1).

The roots of self-directed support

In 1964 Ed Roberts, whose post-polio impairments included quadriplegia and the continuous need for a ventilator to support his breathing, overcame administrative rejection and enrolled as a student of political science at the University of California, Berkeley (Shapiro, 1993). The university housed a small group of students with quadriplegia, who called themselves the rolling quads, in a hospital on the assumption that their substantial impairments required nursing care. Their desire for an ordinary life under their own control, informed by the politics of feminism and civil rights, led to the formation first of the Disabled Students Program at the University and then, in 1971, to the founding of the Center for Independent Living. The Center for Independent Living, an organisation led by disabled people, organised peer support, advocacy, equipment design and

Box 10.1 A note on terminology.

This chapter's vocabulary reflects the way of thinking embodied in the Independent Living movement. We understand *impairments* to be persistent characteristics that affect a person's functioning. Impairments may be evident at birth, they may result from an accident or they may come as a consequence of chronic disease. From this perspective, older people do not require social care because of ageing, but because they acquire impairments in old age. Some impairments require reasonable adjustments to a physical or social setting or individually tailored equipment if the person is to function comfortably and competently there. Some impairments require that the person has effective personal assistance some or all of the time in order to function comfortably and competently in settings that matter to them – whether home, work, leisure or civic life.

On this view, *support for independent living is the key task of social care and a key purpose of health care*. No one is excluded from independent living because of the amount of assistance they require. Independent living does not mean doing everything for yourself; it means having control of the resources you require to enjoy the same substantive freedom everyone expects in order to live the life you wish to lead (Disability Rights Commission, 2006). Such resources may include environmental modifications, equipment and supplies, help with transport, assistance in learning individually chosen skills and personal assistance. Restrictive definitions of personal assistance are unhelpful. It is best understood as 'whatever it takes – that a capable, ethical and well supported assistant can sustainably do – to enable each unique person with impairments to live in a way that makes sense to and for him or her' (see Lyle O'Brien and O'Brien, 1992).

Disability is the disadvantage that people with impairments experience when they encounter barriers to independent living and other opportunities that would otherwise be available to them. Creative action in collaboration with disabled people to remove barriers to full participation in ordinary life and mainstream services is an urgent necessity (Cabinet Office, 2005).

repair, referral to accessible housing, and referral to attendants that people with disabilities could hire with social service funds.

Ed Roberts and other physically disabled activists around the world framed removing the barriers that create disability as a civil rights issue, contested the right of medical and social service practitioners to define their needs or control their lives, lobbied successfully in some places for the capacity to hire and direct their own personal assistants, invented a range of effective supports to allow them to successfully control their own lives and created advocacy and support organisations governed and staffed by disabled people. The way they lived reversed the common understanding of disability that confined people who need personal assistance to their family home or to residential and hospital care.

The elements of self-directed supports

Mrs W (see Box 10.2) participated in Cash & Counseling, a demonstration conducted in three US states between 1999 and 2003 to test the logic of Independent Living for older people and people with developmental disabilities. *Cash* refers to the person's ability to direct the expenditure of an individual allocation of funds and *Counseling* refers to the assistance with planning, problem solving and managing paperwork available to the person and his or her caregivers. The demonstration was evaluated using a random assignment experimental design whose findings support the programme's logic and justify its extension. In comparison to control group members, those who directed their own supports (or whose support was directed by a personal representative, usually a family member) experienced significantly greater satisfaction with their lives and with the assistance they received, and their caregivers reported significantly less burden. Workers reported greater satisfaction with their jobs and with the way they were treated. Involved professionals judged that participants and their representatives ably directed their assistance (Health Services Research, 2007). Although this project was modest in size and restricted in scope, it exemplifies the necessary elements of self-directed supports.

The programme elements that support Mrs W's positive experience are straightforward: she has an *individualised allocation* of funds, based on her assessed need for personal assistance; she has *discretion* in how those funds are spent (e.g. she can choose to save by using somewhat fewer hours of assistance and use the savings to repair her roof); and she has *access to help*, as she requires it, with planning, problem solving and paperwork.

Adopting self-directed support introduces a new system architecture. Typical service architecture responds to population needs by investing in blocks of

---

Box 10.2   Mrs W's story.

Mrs W is an 82-year-old woman who lives alone in a mobile home. Although she is eligible for placement in a nursing home because of physical and sensory impairments consequent to multiple chronic diseases, she wants to remain in her own home. For years she had been dissatisfied with the assistance received through a block-funded home health care agency, so she eagerly enrolled in a programme that offers her control of an individual budget allocation because she values the opportunity to hire her own workers and determine her own priorities. Now, she hires people she knows and trusts to help her according to her directions. She spends a portion of her $100 a week individual budget to buy over-the-counter medications and health care supplies which are not covered by her health insurance. She has also fixed her roof, cleaned her carpet and had her windows washed. 'I couldn't have done any of this myself. I didn't have enough in the bank.' Now, she says, 'I just feel better. I get what I need to get done without much fuss'.

service – various types of residential care, day care, home care – and specifying requirements that providers of these services must meet. People who use such services are one of a group assigned to services to correspond to their assessed need as judged by service system staff variously called case managers, care managers or service coordinators. Self-directed support follows a different design principle: each person who requires personal assistance and those who know and care for him or her are co-producers of the supports a person needs to live as well as he or she can. Money allocated for personal assistance is one resource that a person can combine with other available benefits, resources available to any citizen, and naturally available support to compose a life that makes sense to him or her. Uniform policies govern eligibility and allocation of personal assistance funds; resulting arrangements are various and shift as circumstances and resources do.

This system architecture is analogous to the architecture that allowed IBM to build Blue Gene, the world's fastest and most power-efficient computer as of 2004 (Gara *et al.*, 2005). The design principle spells SMASH: *S*mall, *M*any, and *S*elf-*H*ealing. The system gains its advantage from a very large number of very simple processors working in parallel. This allows the system as a whole to be self-healing: if one path fails, others carry on with the work. Applied to social care, SMASH suggests that the system will increase its effectiveness when it encourages individuals and their allies (1) to make sense of their own changing circumstances; (2) to act within the smallest possible number of system imposed constraints to pursue goals that they define as desirable; (3) to learn from and connect with others as they choose. This requires that system managers refrain from predetermining such matters as how many people will live together or what range of supports, activities and therapies will be available to members of a served group.

Benefits and common objections

The social space opened and supported by discretion in directing an individual allocation with help available enables Mrs W to mobilise the resources available to her to live a life that makes sense to her as she incorporates impairment into her life's narrative. As she notes, these resources combine in richer and more complex and interesting ways than those available to her from typical service provision. In addition to her allocation and what it buys, her resources include trust in those she chooses to assist her; the self-efficacy she feels in exercising her decision-making powers to select goals and engaging her capacities to work towards them (Bandura, 2002); the security evoked by a sense of fit between the assistance she prefers and the assistance she receives; the continuity she experiences with familiar places and people; and the satisfaction she derives from saving and spending to improve her living circumstances and her modest material legacy.

Seasoned service managers may react to this apparent good news with caution. Workers might exploit Mrs W's trust. Mrs W might make bad decisions that lead to a deterioration in her health. Mrs W might increase risk by saving on hours of help, and anyway, if she can manage with fewer hours of assistance, shouldn't her allocation be reduced? Mrs W might live in a rundown place with awful neighbours she would be better away from. Auditors or elected members might view Mrs W's roof repairs as an illegitimate use of public funds. Mrs W herself might fiddle the programme and find a way to buy cigarettes and lottery tickets with the funds. And anyway, Mrs W is the capable exception to the dependent, incompetent, confused and passive clientele that typically demand services. The vulnerability that people who require personal assistance cope with and their human fallibility are incontestable. However, assumptions about how best to address these realities are worth debating.

Existing services have not solved the highlighted problems. Organised professional bureaucracies, whether publicly or privately operated, have not eliminated the risks enumerated above, even at the cost of substantial expenditures and demanding serious trade-offs in personal autonomy. Thus, costs for Cash & Counseling were somewhat higher than those for controls because participants were able to hire people who actually delivered the number of hours of service authorised, whereas the agencies that served control group members could not or did not deliver planned and authorised amounts of service (Dale and Brown, 2007). In the same way, the precipitous decrease in autonomy required by moving into a staff-controlled residential setting is no guarantee of competence in even the most basic health and safety-related tasks: about half of care homes and nursing homes in England fail when assessed against standards designed to assure that people receive the right dosages of the right medications at the right time, and this despite focused inspection effort, guidance, support and training (Commission for Social Care Inspection, 2006). As a final example, an organisation operating a licensed and inspected, not-for-profit care home defrauded the state of New York by improperly billing for more than $800 000 in undelivered professional services over a 5-year period, despite one of the world's most elaborate and expensive accounting requirements and fraud detection units (NYS Commission on Quality of Care, 2001).

Worries about misuse of money increase costs. The biggest demand on the counsellors available to participants in Cash & Counseling, and the most common cause of delay in initiating services, was the paperwork required to hedge against the possibility that the initiative would be seen to be unaccountable for public funds. In fact, extremely little misuse of funds occurred (Mahoney *et al.*, 2007). This is not an argument against reasonable accountability, but a reminder that transaction costs are driven up by managers' concerns about punishment and unfavourable media or political attention falling on them. These concerns express and increase suspicion that most users of personal assistance are untrustworthy or that public and political support for social care in community settings is so shallow and unstable that its very existence could be threatened (on the perception of low public support for social care and some of its consequences, see Platt, 2007).

Paternalism is not free. The assumption that service workers and managers know better than people and families requiring assistance remains dominant in practice, though its rhetorical power has decreased. National policy directives promise that people will soon have greater choice, a much louder voice and greater responsibility in the services they receive – a promise that implies radical change in the mindsets, relationships and practices that define the current system (Department of Health, 2006). For this strategy to work, people who use services will need to assume new roles and accept new responsibilities, from adopting healthy patterns of exercise and eating, to assuming greater self-management of chronic disease as expert patients. The health system cannot afford passive patients, nor can the personal assistance system afford passive consumers. The paternalistic mindset that assumes that people who require personal assistance are incompetent and untrustworthy until they prove otherwise drives two unacceptable and mutually reinforcing costs. It embeds a disrespectful attitude in the foundation of social care and normalises practices that mindlessly compromise people's rights, such as the routine shunting of people into residential care for lack of investment in sufficient alternative supports (Disability Rights Commission, 2006). It too often encourages, or even requires, the passivity that justifies it. This results in losses of opportunity and life quality, the extent of which is unknown and unknowable (Deming, 2000).

Uncertainties should be resolved with bold tests. Environmental pressure on social care grows inexorably. More people survive for much longer with impairments that require personal assistance. The ratio of younger earners to older pensioners decreases. The supply of people who choose to work as paid personal assistants declines. More families live at a distance or pursue work lives whose time demands make caregiving increasingly difficult. Fewer neighbourhoods have norms that support informal care. Service providers, from general practitioners and social workers to postal carriers, juggle greater demand and more requirements, most predicated on the assumptions that more can be done with less and that better quality will follow automatically from imposing more demanding targets from above. In public services, reorganisation has itself become a significant transaction cost when the adjustment time of involved people is accounted for. Many people remain uncertain about the entitlements and duties of citizenship, but there is a sense of disappointed expectation and resentment around many public services. Public money seems overcommitted, family members seem overcommitted, service staff seem overcommitted. In this environment it is uncertain how many Mrs Ws there are, how effectively and accountably they or those who know them will be able to self-direct necessary assistance, how much they will be able to mobilise other resources, and how much of what kind of publicly funded assistance they will need to accomplish all this. Uncertainty can rationalise going on as usual or taking tiny, timid steps. It should signal the urgency of bold actions that can generate deeper knowledge and greater capacity. The test of partnership working is the motivation the partnership draws from its participants to take and learn from bold steps that respect and support citizen capacities.

Learning from experience

Andre's experience in Box 10.3 demonstrates that the elements of self-directed support – discretion over an individual allocation with necessary help – can

> **Box 10.3**   Andre's story.
>
> Andre is in his mid-20s and capably does government office work that has been customised to make the most of his abilities, which are shaped by substantial cognitive, physical and language impairments. He greatly enjoys swimming, the outdoors and travel. He lives in his own home, which he shares with a married couple who work as his paid assistants and their daughter. Like the other 1250 people served by his county's Developmental Disabilities Program, Andre has an individual budget, which in his case is directed for him by his mother, who is his legal guardian. She has chosen to take primary responsibility for hiring, training, scheduling and supervising his personal assistants and coordinating with the employment support organisations that assist Andre on the job and with his health care providers. Both Andre and his mother are helped to deal with programme requirements by an independent service broker (in this case a friend who volunteers his time) and supported by a circle of unpaid people whom they have chosen and trust for counsel and for occasional practical help.

sustain complex and intensive personal assistance for a person whose cognitive and communication impairments require a substitute decision-maker. His county, a participant in a US national demonstration project aimed at implementing self-determination as an option for people with developmental disabilities (Bradley *et al.*, 2001; Rossiter and Harkins, 2005), shows that a whole local system can be transformed to and managed through self-directed support.

Andre is not typical of the people who use personal assistance services in his county, though the innovations that have grown up to support him have influenced expectations among people who rely on services and practices among service agencies. He is among the most impaired of the people the county serves and his family and support circle are among the most active, both in day-to-day management and in the amount of scheduled unpaid assistance they offer. (About 5% of the total number of people the county serves choose to self-manage service budgets as Andre's mother does; others negotiate with service providers to organise and manage more of what they require, while many people simply select the offering that suits them from among available service providers.) Most people who require as much assistance as Andre does live with one or two disabled roommates with the assistance of a supported living programme. Most people and substitute decision-makers also use their budgets to select the service organisations with whom they and their brokers negotiate an individualised support plan. Some substitute decision-makers disapprove of changes that service providers who know and also care about the person think would be desirable, and some people have conflicts with family members about what they want to do. Some families are disengaged, especially when a person was placed in residential care as a child or young person, and some are unable to be involved much (often because they are themselves experiencing impairments as they have aged or because they are providing unpaid care to other family members with impairments). A few families attempt to exploit the system and have been replaced as substitute decision-makers. And a small number of family members are neglectful or abusive of the person, often because they are themselves affected by addiction or mental ill health and come to the attention of protective services or the courts.

Andre's county has myriad quality issues to engage and faces the same sorts of environmental pressures that any other overcommitted system does. There are also ethical questions that come more sharply into view with self-direction. The supply of good quality services is stretched, and a number of people would prefer services from a provider who does not have spare capacity to accept them. Some believe that it is wrong for family investment to count for as much difference in living conditions as it does for people like Andre. Some are suspicious that substitute

---

Box 10.4   International examples.

Within the UK there are at least three different approaches to self-directed support: the Independent Living Fund, Direct Payments and in Control's system that include the concept of an individual budget.

Within the US there are numerous initiatives and there are significant variations within these models, not only between states, but also at the level of the county. Moreover, there are many such systems in other countries:

- Germany's social insurance scheme enables people to take their funding as cash.
- France's *Prestation Spécifique Dépendance* gives cash to disabled people for support.
- Austria has an individualised funding programme called Cash Allowance for Care.
- There are several Canadian initiatives, for example, the Individualised Quality of Life Project in Ontario.
- There are some Australian programmes, for example, Future for Young Adults in Victoria.
- New Zealand has an individualised funding programme.
- In Sweden the Personal Assistance Act created a system of direct funding for support.
- In the Netherlands there is a system of personal budgets (*'persoosgebonden budget'*).

To date, most schemes tend to have a limited focus: some serve older people while others are just for younger adults. People with learning difficulties are often excluded altogether. This tendency to limit approaches to service-defined labels has the impact of reinforcing traditional, system-focused models of care delivery.

See, e.g., Halloran, 1998; Glasby and Littlechild, 2002; Robbins, 2006.

decision makers, especially parents, will not take adequate account of the person's own interests and desires. Some advocates for particular approaches to service are concerned that self-direction offers too little protection against what they see as undesirable practice or too little incentive to provide what they believe people really need. Self-directed supports do not dissolve quality issues or resolve ethical questions. Indeed, the contrasts that emerge as people make different decisions about their lives and the ways that personal assistance fits in make some of these issues and questions occasions for learning.

What Andre's county has done is shift the context for development. The elements of self-directed support provide the mechanism, but the change springs from a change in mindset. Most social care systems act as if they assumed that the typical people and families who rely on them for personal assistance are incompetent, self-interested to the point that they will exploit the system in any way that is open to them, and inferior in the exercise of judgement to social care staff. The system that assists Andre begins with the opposite assumptions and manages the conflicts that arise from occasional poor judgement, excessive self-interest, incompetence, neglect and abuse as exceptions that deserve intensive attention from county staff. These staff have more time to discover and attend to exceptions because most people and their families are managing the services they use to their satisfaction and within applicable rules. This is one example of a particular type of self-directed support, Box 10.4 outlines other international examples which are not covered in detail within this chapter which are in place in a range of different countries (see Box 10.4).

From option to operating system

In the UK Gavin and his family and friends organise his support in a locality that is learning how to transform its social care system by implementing in Control, a comprehensive way to generate self-directed supports that functions like an open-source operating system does for a computer network (see Box 10.5). Most other

---

Box 10.5   Gavin's story.

In his late 30s, Gavin's mobility, swallowing, speech and vision became significantly impaired consequent to multiple sclerosis. As he made his self-directed support plan, he stated his purpose: 'living my life my way, with the love and support of my family and friends'. Gavin's family and friends provide sufficient unpaid natural support to allow him to spend significantly less than his full allocated individual budget. He buys paid personal assistance, laundry and ironing, reflexology and a season football ticket (an expenditure that generates 4 hours a week of free personal assistance in season, which is worth more than 2.5 times the cost of the ticket). A colleague handles payroll at a cost of 'one Thai green curry per month'. (See a video version of Gavin's support plan at http://www.picturethispartnership.org.uk)

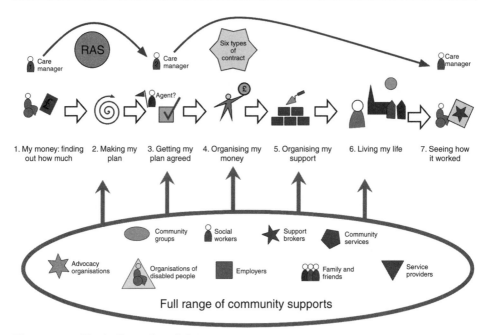

Figure 10.2 The in Control model.

approaches offer self-directed support as one option for clients approved by the system and restrict clients to particular means (e.g. people can only direct particular services or buy from preselected providers; people must use an approved broker to prepare a plan or use a fiscal intermediary to manage their funds). in Control is comprehensive in that it re-orients the whole system to self-directed supports by making all funds for assistance liquid and specifying a sequence of necessary steps to implement support, each of which citizens can choose to perform in a variety of legitimate ways (see Figure 10.2) in order to access and expend their individual budget. in Control is like an operating system in that it is a set of policies, practices and tools that allow local authorities to convert policy demands for greater per-sonalisation and choice into practical means to meet citizen demands for support legally and flexibly. in Control is open source in that it publishes its policies and tools on its website (see http://www.in-control.org.uk), invites use and revision, and incorporates improvements as they are endorsed by its editorial board (an expert group representing its 16-partner organisations).

The variety of individual capacities and preferences in a local population calls for many options. People unable to make or communicate judgements without assistance can be represented by a personal agent. There are at least six ways to hold and disburse funds. People who want assistance in making a support plan and negotiating for services can engage a broker. People who want to hire and supervise their own staff can do so; people who want to purchase a service that packages assistance can do so, and so on.

Gavin's contract with the social care system is based on a shared appreciation of the rights and responsibilities of citizenship, not on a professionally controlled definition of the appropriate service response to his system defined needs. Accountability for public funds demands that his eligibility for social care be officially certified, the amount of social care funding allocated to him be administered through a fair and transparent resource allocation system (step 1 in Figure 10.2), and that his expenditures be legal and open to audit. Within these limits, he and his family and friends are free to set goals, prioritise resource use, determine means and pursue a life that make sense to them. In doing so he creates social exchanges based on mutual regard (Thai curry for payroll services), economic exchanges (laundry and ironing by someone local) and links to other publicly funded resources (Access to Work employment support funding). Gavin is not a consumer but a citizen, co-producing the supports required to 'live my life my way'. in Control supports him to experience assistance in the context of his individual interests and struggles rather than to compromise individuality and choice in order to receive the assistance that someone at a professional distance deems good for him.

Developing a shared understanding of citizenship calls for a shift in mindset by those who require assistance as well as those who manage and provide social care. Many people hold an unexamined assumption that need for assistance suspends the responsibilities of citizenship and puts the person in the passive role of client, one taken care of by state agents who should be responsible for doing what is best. This belief is in tension with people's desire for autonomy, a tension which in Control seeks to resolve by rooting all of its efforts in a clear understanding of citizenship.

This understanding identifies six interacting keys to citizenship which put support in context (Duffy, 2003). Support is one key for every citizen, and assistance funded by an individual social care budget is one possible means of support for eligible citizens with impairments. The six keys to citizenship are the following:

- *Self-determination* – making our own decisions, being in control of our life
- *Direction* – having a meaningful life that suits us and the kind of unique individuals that we are
- *Money* – being able to pay our way and to decide how we will meet our own needs
- *Home* – having a place of our own, where we are safe, where we belong
- *Support* – getting help, when we need it, to do the things we really want to do
- *Community life* – playing an active part in our family, our circle of friends and our community

These six values of citizenship specify the outcomes of an adequate system of social care. These outcomes are most likely when all the actors in a local system continually improve their ability to reflect these principles in their interactions with each other (see Table 10.1).

Table 10.1   Key principles of self-directed support.

Principles	Meaning
1. Right to independent living – *I can get the support I need to be an independent citizen*	If someone has an impairment which means they need help to fulfil their role as a citizen, then they should get the help they need
2. Right to a personalised budget – *I know how much money I can use for my support*	If someone needs ongoing paid help as part of their life, they should be able to decide how the money that pays for that help is used
3. Right to self-determination – *I have the authority, support or representation to make my own decisions*	If someone needs help to make decisions then decision-making should be made as close to the person as possible, reflecting the person's own interests and preferences
4. Right to accessibility – *I can understand the rules and systems and am able to get help easily*	The system of rules within which people have to work must be clear and open in order to maximise the ability of the disabled person to take control of their own support
5. Right to flexible funding – *I can use my money flexibly and creatively*	When someone is using their personalised budget, they should be free to spend their funds in the way that makes best sense to them, without unnecessary restrictions
6. Accountability principle – *I should tell people how I used my money and anything I have learnt*	The disabled person and the government both have a responsibility to each other to explain their decisions and to share what they have learnt
7. Capacity principle – *give me enough help, but not too much; I have got something to contribute too*	Disabled people, their families and their communities must not be assumed to be incapable of managing their own support, learning skills and making a contribution

Discussion and conclusion: a new framework for partnership

As various chapters in this text demonstrate, partnership working to date has tended to be conceived as a partnership between agencies who are expected to find ways of actively collaborating in order that the different services they offer are better integrated. The citizen is, probably rightly, supposed not to be interested in the organisational boundaries that define those agencies nor the precise definition of their core roles. However, it is challenging to expect those agencies to collaborate when, by definition, their core business will be distinct (e.g. local authorities responsible for social care will, whatever the overlap, be focused on different citizens, different needs, different professional groups, different accountabilities). The rhetoric of partnership cannot put together what politics and organisational design have put asunder.

In contrast, self-directed support offers a different way of approaching this problem. Instead of focusing the task of partnership at the level of the agency, it suggests that the primary focus must be on a partnership with the citizen. The primary reason why this approach may well be more effective is that most support is already offered by family, friends or members of the wider community. The primary focus of integration for the citizen will be on integrating resources or support from agencies with these community supports, but this can only happen at the level of the citizen and requires the citizen to have meaningful control of the resources that the agencies provide. In fact, one can sharpen this point further and argue that organisational simplification, integration or alliance may even risk reducing the possible leverage that the citizen has over the citizen. The ideal of a 'one-stop shop' supposes that the shop has something you can buy and something you want to buy, but if what you want cannot be bought or what is on offer does not suit you, then limiting the offering of agencies will limit and distort the citizen's options.

As a result, the energy that is currently deployed to achieve system integration may be better used to strengthen the citizen's ability to achieve personalised integration. This will enhance genuine partnership working in at least four ways:

- A shared understanding of citizenship and the principles for organising support that flow from understanding the needs for the deep changes necessary to respond to a turbulent environment shaped by changing demographics, developing technologies and changing political, economic and social conditions. The practical sense of citizenship that animates in Control provides a foundation for the dialogue necessary to establish this orientation.
- Recognition of the power of designing systems that contain complexity in small, multiple, and self-healing units of action can reduce the load on more hierarchal forms of organisation, especially when much necessary coordination can be exercised by units as small and connected as the people and families who require support and their allies. The experience of self-directed support suggests that much more is possible in this direction than has so far been realised.
- Redrawing those dysfunctional boundaries that generate the demand for integration, while at the same time creating disincentives to it, would considerably ease the strains on partnership work. Most notably, the UK's distinction between health and social care breaks down as soon as people move away from acute care and begin to cope with impairments to functioning. The political issues in redefining boundaries to put all of the non-acute health and social care resources available to support people with impairments into a unified entitlement to self-directed supports are daunting. The likely improvement in citizenship outcomes makes it worth struggling for.
- Many of the greatest benefits to citizens with impairments will come within the boundaries of departments, levels of government and agencies rather then across them. Mainstream services and markets that are accessible and willing to learn how to make reasonable adjustments to the requirements of citizens with impairments are easier for people to join up for themselves than they are for managers to join up by command at distant points. This shortens the agenda for partnerships by reducing the number of inter-organisational boundaries to contest and defend.

Within the UK, the journey towards a meaningful, citizenship-based account of integration has only just begun. Early initiatives have come from the world of social care and particularly from those people involved in the Independent Living movement. One sign that these changes can begin to influence the health care system is the recent announcement of a joint health and social programme in Barnsley which they call *Every Adult Matters*. Their vision is to see 'people maximise their aspirations for control and independence over their health and well-being supported by flexible, responsive, preventative services' (Barnsley Council and Barnsley PCT, 2007). This kind of approach may be the first sign of a radically more realistic approach to partnership working.

Summary

- Adopting the principles of the Independent Living movement can lead to a different perspective on the challenges of integration.
- Systems of self-directed support are beginning to offer individuals much greater control over the shape of their own support.
- Early evidence from many different countries suggests that self-directed support is more effective at achieving positive outcomes for people than more bureaucratic systems.
- The new system architecture for self-directed support suggests that people will want services to offer more choice and flexibility rather than integration and standardisation.
- Some countries, particularly the UK, are starting to explore the possibility of a universal system transformation across all services for disabled people.
- These new approaches may suggest that our current focus on organisational integration may need to be reconsidered as people develop citizen-centred solutions to integration.

Further reading and useful websites

Useful sources include:

Duffy, S. (2003) *Keys to Citizenship*. Birkenhead, Paradigm.

Leadbeater, C. *et al.* (2008) *Making It Personal*. London, Demos.

Poll, C. and Duffy, S. (eds.) (2008) *A Report on in Control's Second Phase 2006–2007*, in London, Control Publications.

Poll, C. *et al.* (2006) *A Report on in Control's First Phase 2003–2005*, in London, Control Publications.

Relevant websites include:

Cash & Counseling: http://www.cashandcounseling.org/

Dane County, Wisconsin Human Services describes the programmes, policies and procedures through which the county administers self-directed services: http://www.dane-countyhumanservices.org/disability.htm

in Control: http://www.in-control.org.uk/

UK Office for Disability Issues: http://www.officefordisability.gov.uk/

World Institute on Disability: http://www.wid.org/

References

Bandura, A. (2002) *Self-Efficacy in Changing Societies*. Cambridge, Cambridge University Press.

Barnsley Council and PCT (2007) *Every Adult Matters*. Barnsley, Barnsley MBC and Barnsley PCT.

Bradley, V. *et al.* (2001) *The Robert Wood Johnson Foundation Self-Determination Initiative: Final Impact Assessment Report*. Cambridge, MA, Human Services Research Institute.

Cabinet Office (2005) *Improving the Life Chances of Disabled People*. London, Prime Minister's Strategy Unit.

CSCI (2006) *Handle with Care: Managing Medications for Residents of Care Homes and Children's Homes – A Follow-Up Study*. London, Commission for Social Care Inspection.

Dale, S. and Brown, R. (2007) How does cash and counseling affect costs? *Health Services Research*, 42(1, pt 2), 488–509.

Deming, W.E. (2000) *The New Economics for Industry, Government, Education*, 2nd edn. Cambridge, MA, MIT Press.

Department of Health (2006) *Our Health, Our Care, Our Say: A New Direction for Community Services*. London, HMSO.

Disability Rights Commission (2006) *Independent Living Discussion Paper*. London, Disability Rights Commission.

Duffy, S. (2003) *Keys to Citizenship*. Birkenhead, Paradigm.

Duffy, S. (2004) *In Control*, Journal of Integrated Care, December 2004 Volume 12 issue 6.

Gara, A. *et al.* (2005) Overview of the Blue Gene/L system architecture, *IBM Journal of Research and Development*, 49(2–3), 195–212.

Glasby, J. and Littlechild, R. (2002) *Social Work and Direct Payments*. Bristol, Policy Press.

Halloran, J. (ed.) (1998) *Towards a People's Europe: A Report on the Development of Direct Payments in 10 Member States of the European Union*. Vienna, European Social Network.

Health Services Research (2007) Special issue: putting consumers first in long-term care – findings from the Cash & Counseling demonstration and evaluation, *Health Services Research*, 42(1, pt 2), 353–586.

Lyle O'Brien, C. and O'Brien, J. (1992) *A Checklist for Evaluating Personal Assistance Policies and Programs*. Syracuse, NY, The Center on Human Policy. Available online via http://thechp.syr.edu/pas.pdf

Mahoney, K. *et al.* (2007) The future of cash and counseling: the framers' view, *Health Services Research*, 42(1, pt 2), 550–566.

NYS Commission on Quality of Care (2001) *Exploiting Not-for-Profit Care in an Adult Home: The Story Behind Ocean House Center*. Albany, NY, New York State Commission on Quality of Care for the Mentally Disabled.

Platt, D. (2007) *The Status of Social Care: A Review*. London, Department of Health.

Robbins, D. (2006) *Choice, Control and Individual Budgets: Emerging Themes*. London, Social Care Institute for Excellence.

Rossiter, D. and Harkins, D. (2005) *Forging a Partnership: Individualizing Funding and Increasing Choices for People with Developmental Disabilities*. Madison, WI, Dane County Human Services.

Shapiro, J.P. (1993) *No Pity*. New York, Times Books.

11 The outcomes of health and social care partnerships

Helen Dickinson

The past 30 years has witnessed an international trend of governments becoming increasingly interested in the outcomes which their services produce and at what costs. This propensity is generally associated with the paradigm of new public management (NPM) (see the Introduction to this book for further detail). As Hood (1991) describes, NPM is characterised by an increased decentralisation of power to local levels with managers increasingly taking responsibility for budgets and being allowed greater flexibilities in terms of their actions, but simultaneously bearing more responsibility for the outputs and outcomes of that particular unit.

So far, the majority of contributions to this text have been more concerned with the means, rather than the ends of partnership working. In other words, most chapters have demonstrated greater interest in how health and social care partnerships might be made to operate more effectively together and less with the impact which these working relationships might have on service users. This is not necessarily just a quirk of this book, but is representative of a much wider trend in terms of health and social care partnership research. Implicit in many of these conceptualisations is the notion that by health and social care organisations working together effectively in partnership – however difficult that task might be – it will improve outcomes for individuals who use these services. As this book has demonstrated, health and social care partnerships are viewed as important mechanisms for improving service delivery throughout much of the developed world and in theory promise much. Yet, in practice, the empirical data to demonstrate this improvement has often proved elusive, with a number of commentators noting that partnerships have so far failed to demonstrate a significant impact on service user outcomes (e.g. Brown *et al.*, 2003; Kharicha *et al.*, 2004; Townsley *et al.*, 2004; Davey *et al.*, 2005). This chapter aims to explore issues surrounding the evaluation of partnerships, particularly in terms of the impact which they might have on service user outcomes, and argues that this lack of evidence may, in part, be a result of the scale of the evaluation challenge – rather than a lack of impact per se.

The chapter starts by exploring definitions of key terms surrounding outcomes, before moving on to give a brief overview of the difficulties inherent in evaluating the outcomes of partnership working. It then proceeds to analyse a range of examples of international partnership evaluations and the types of impacts these studies have demonstrated. The chapter concludes with a series of key lessons from these examples and the implications for the evaluation of partnerships.

What are outcomes?

Historically, health and social care services tended to be evaluated in terms of re-source inputs (how much they spent), activities (what they did) and outputs (what they produced). However, partly influenced by NPM and a general trend for gov-ernments to become more cost-effective and transparent in their actions, public sector organisations are increasingly seeking to demonstrate the actual impact of their services – rather than just the volume or number of activities carried out. Out-puts are direct products or services which stem from the activities of a particular initiative and are delivered to a target group, but they are unable to demonstrate quality of services. Outcomes differ from outputs as they are the total external con-sequences of services or initiatives delivered, rather than simply the products. For example, the numbers of older people in residential care or living independently in a specified period refer to outputs, but they say little about whether the life of these older people is good or bad relative to the norm. Nicholas and colleagues (2003) define an outcome as the total 'impact, effect or consequence of help received' (p. 2). This broad definition is illustrative of what Smith (1996) argues is the very specific connotation which outcomes in the public sector have: namely, the 'impact on society of a particular public sector activity' (p. 1). In other words, the purpose of measuring outcomes in the public sector is about assessing the valuation we place on an activity.

As indicated in the introductory section to this chapter a range of commenta-tors have noted that health and social care partnerships are yet to unequivocally demonstrate that they impact upon service user outcomes. However, as Dowling *et al.* (2004) note, the picture may be slightly more nuanced than this suggests. The authors note that partnership evaluations have tended to be more concerned with issues of *process* than of *outcomes*. That is, they have tended to focus on organisa-tional factors (how effectively partners are working together), rather than whether these working arrangements have in fact impacted on the services delivered or the outcomes of individuals receiving services. This interest in process may sim-ply be a reflection that the assumption that partnerships lead to better outcomes is so engrained within the public sector (and evaluators' beliefs) that rather than investigating service user outcomes, evaluators analyse the process of partnership working, and if this seems smooth, presume that positive benefits are being pro-duced for service users. If we accept the rhetoric that partnerships lead to better service user outcomes, then simply evaluating how partners work together should give us an indication of whether the partnership is having a positive impact.

However, this preoccupation with process issues may also be indicative of the difficulties associated with selecting which outcome indicators to use in demon-strating the impact of partnership working. As Dowling and colleagues (2004) fur-ther note, the aims of partnerships are often similar to those of other public sector policies (i.e. improved efficiency and effectiveness). Therefore, demonstrating what it is specifically that partnerships aim to achieve outside of traditional modes of service delivery might be problematic. Drawing on evidence from the US, Schmitt (2001) suggests what is often missing from evaluations of collaborative efforts is an explanation of *why* certain outcome indicators were selected. These studies often lack a clear rationale behind the selection of outcome indicators, with some being selected for ease of use, rather than necessarily because they are the most appropriate. As different types of partnerships might aim to achieve very different things, it is important that the most appropriate outcome indicators are selected for that partnership – and these may differ from outcomes associated with other partnerships.

In recent years the UK government has aimed to be more explicit about the outcomes it is aiming to achieve through its public services. It is proposed that adult services should be working towards the following outcomes (Department of Health, 2006; see HM Treasury, 2003, for outcomes for children's services):

- Improved health and emotional well-being
- Improved quality of life
- Making a positive contribution
- Choice and control
- Freedom from discrimination
- Economic well-being
- Personal dignity

Within this context, health and social care organisations should be working together to try and influence these outcomes. However, evaluating these outcomes will clearly be a much more complex task than measuring outputs (e.g. the numbers of individuals accessing specific services). These outcomes are multifaceted and may be affected by a wide range of variables beyond the remit of partner organisations. For this reason, the New Zealand government guidance on performance management (Treasury and State Services Commission, 2007) suggests outcomes might be broken down into near-term results, intermediate results and end outcomes. (This approach is also taken by the Office of the Auditor General of Canada, 2003.) This perspective suggests that intervention logics should underpin all public sector activities, with organisations having a clear sense of what the end result of any activity should be – in addition to the intermediate steps which will lead to this point and any potential external activities which might confound potential impact (see Figure 11.1 for illustration).

This approach is broadly similar to 'Theories of Change' (Connell *et al.*, 1995; Fulbright-Anderson *et al.*, 1998) which seeks to surface all the theories underpinning how and why a programme will work in as fine detail as possible and identify all the assumptions and sub-assumptions built in to a programme or intervention. It is a 'systematic and cumulative study of the links between activities, outcomes and contexts of the initiative' (Connell and Kubisch, 1998, p. 18). According to this perspective, evaluations should seek to demonstrate which of the assumptions

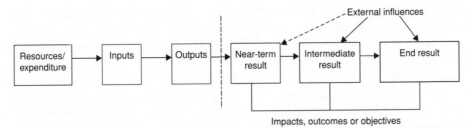

Figure 11.1   Intervention logic. (From Treasury and State Services Commission, 2007, p. 5.)

underlying a programme break down, where they collapse and which of the several theories behind the programme are best supported by the evidence (Weiss, 1995). Having surfaced all the assumptions and short-, intermediate- and long-term outcomes, a programme or intervention is thought to be able to influence or deliver, selecting which outcomes to measure should be a relatively simple task.

One final issue of note in terms of defining outcomes is that Beresford *et al.* (2000) suggest that the way in which services are delivered may have an important bearing on service user outcomes. Whilst service users are concerned that services will help them achieve the outcomes they aspire to, they are also concerned that services are delivered in ways which empower rather than disempower. In this way, Nicholas *et al.* (2003) differentiate *service process* as one type of outcome. Service process outcomes reflect the impact of the way in which services are delivered, for example, being treated as a human being; feeling that privacy and confidentiality are respected; and being treated as someone with a right to services. What this suggests is that the process of service delivery cannot easily be divorced from the impact it produces; the mode of service delivery may be integral to the delivery of certain outcomes.

Challenges of partnership evaluation

There are a range of difficulties and complexities which partnership evaluations might encounter (some of which are also true of other evaluations of complex policy initiatives). A more full account of these issues may be found elsewhere (Glendinning, 2002; Hudson and Hardy, 2002; Dickinson, 2006), but this section is intended to outline the main problems that pertain to the identification and measurement of outcomes. One of the primary difficulties relates to the many different forms which health and social care partnerships might take. As other chapters in this book illustrate, partnerships may look very different in practice and it is likely that most are intended to achieve different ends. Consequently, it is difficult to draw out generalisable lessons about 'partnerships' and outcomes.

However, it is not just differences between partnerships which might be of concern. Partnerships are often composed of a number of groups who may have quite different perspectives of what it should achieve and of how the partnership should be evaluated (Thomas and Palfrey, 1996). Although partners will likely have some common goal in terms of the partnership, outside of this initial aim they may have quite different objectives. One of the difficulties of adopting a Theories of Change approach is that different stakeholders will often have different percep- tions of what constitutes success for a partnership (Barnes *et al.*, 2005). Thus, a primary complexity in evaluating partnerships lies in determining a consensus be- tween partners in terms of what the outcomes will look like if the partnership is successful. Moreover, even if a partnership reaches consensus between all its con- stituent partners about what success would constitute, it does not necessarily follow that service users will share this vision. Failure to recognise different concepts of success leads to inappropriate conclusions about the effectiveness of partnerships and potentially to the inappropriate application of research results (Ouwens *et al.*, 2005).

A further difficulty which partnership evaluations often encounter is the issue of attribution. As the previous section suggested, the aims of partnerships are often broadly similar to those of other improvement initiatives. Isolating the impact of a partnership can be challenging: particularly when aiming to affect changes in broad outcomes, it can be difficult to demonstrate that it was the actions of the partnership which caused this change and not any other factors. This process is made even more complex given that partnerships are often established to tackle 'wicked' or endemic problems embedded within local communities. It may take some time to impact upon these issues, or we may only see the impact of actions after a significant time lag. As such, the influence of partnership working may be subtle, indirect and cumulative – rather than a direct reflection of a programme. However, adopting a Theories of Change or intervention logic approach as outlined earlier might, to some degree, overcome difficulties of attribution. By being clear about what it is that a partnership is aiming to achieve and by what means, it may prove easier to attribute particular outcomes to a partnership.

The final point of note for this section concerns the issue of process. As outlined earlier, partnership evaluations have had a tendency to concentrate more on the process of partnership working than on outcomes. However, to simply measure outcomes without acknowledging the context for the partnership, or how well partners are interacting, may not give a full picture of the nature of the partnership. Again, as illustrated by the Theories of Change approach, if a partnership is not functioning effectively then it may not lead to the expected impacts. For example, Davey *et al.* (2005) demonstrate how the co-location of health and social care teams had little impact over their interaction and did not necessarily lead to closer working as had originally been predicted. Clearly this has important connotations for any potential impact that this way of working was intended to produce. Although an evaluation may be primarily concerned with any impact on service user outcomes, it will be necessary to do some form of process evaluation to check these causal links. Without examining process, an evaluation is doing little more than inferring causation from the input and outcomes of a partnership. Failure to look inside this 'black box' (Robson, 1993) means that it is difficult to say with confidence which parts of the programme worked and why, whether they would be applicable to different situations and if there are any positive or negative effects which would otherwise not be anticipated (Birckmayer and Weiss, 2000).

What does the international evidence tell us about evaluating partnerships?

As suggested by the previous section, evaluating service user outcomes of partnerships is a complex task. One possibility, therefore, is that the lack of unequivocal evidence linking partnerships to service user outcomes might be an expression of this complexity, rather than a lack of impact per se. This section investigates this link by analysing the impacts which a range of international examples of partnership working have been demonstrated to achieve.

Clinical and functional indicators

There are several examples of partnership evaluation which have sought to examine functional or clinical indicators of individuals using services and link changes to the activities of partnerships. However, just as the professions and procedures of health and social care have developed separately, so too have their outcome indicators. There are substantially more health-related outcomes in comparison with those connected to social care (Nocon and Qureshi, 1996), and the nature of these outcome indicators varies according to their differing conceptualisations of health and well-being. Whilst social care outcomes are traditionally wider in perspective and concerned with everyday aspects of life, medical indicators are predominantly allied with 'negative' (i.e. disease-free) views of health and tend to be associated with clinical indicators embedded in the quantitative approach (Young and Chesson, 2006). Moreover, unlike health outcomes, the majority of social care is about maintaining a level, rather than making specific improvements in user's lives. Qureshi *et al.* (1998) estimate that around 85% of social care work is directed at sustaining a level of an acceptable quality of life. Thus, many of the indicators which broadly come under this heading tend to link more to health than social care services and as such will be more applicable to some types of partnership arrangements than others.

There are a range of examples within the partnership literature (predominantly linked to integrated care for older people) which have been evaluated for their impact on clinical and functional indicators. A number of these studies found that partnership working had no statistically significant impact on clinical indicators or positive impact on functional levels of service users (e.g. Brown *et al.*, 2003; Davey *et al.*, 2005). One such example is Hultberg *et al.*'s (2002, 2005) evaluation of an interdisciplinary musculoskeletal disorder project in Sweden. The research team found very little difference in health status between patients under the co-financed system compared to the control groups. However, the team note, 'the optimal design to test effectiveness is a randomized controlled trial, which was not possible in this study since it was an observational assessment of a natural experiment ... We had difficulties including the desired number of patients and the small sample size gave the study low statistical power' (Hultberg *et al.*, 2005, pp. 121–122). Thus, there were difficulties in this case with the type of evaluation approach which was possible given the context. The team also state that they did not know if the co-financed teams actually changed the way in which services were delivered and had not been able to analyse these actions within this research project. Clearly this has implications for any potential lessons that might be learned about specific aspects of partnership working and implications which these might have for service users.

Many of these projects are set up to aid individuals with chronic and complex problems, and so, in a number of ways, expecting to see significant impacts on clinical and functional outcomes might perhaps be unrealistic. Yet, despite this, some evaluations have shown impacts on these factors. Thus, the On Lok project in the US (see Eng *et al.*, 1997, for an overview; see also Chapters 3, 5 and 8) also found significant improvement in a variety of functional indicators. Yordi and Waldman (1985) suggest that this programme helped individuals develop compensatory skills to adjust and cope with their impairments, rather than being able to reverse these conditions. The Canadian PRISMA (Programme of Research to Integrate Services for the Maintenance of Autonomy) programme (see Hébert *et al.*, 2005, and Chapter 5 for an overview) found some evidence of maintenance of service users' functional autonomy, although this dropped off significantly in the third year of the project (Tourigny *et al.*, 2004). Similarly, the Vittorio Veneto and Rovereto projects in Italy demonstrated improvements on several functional measures for individuals receiving integrated care compared with control groups (Bernabei *et al.*, 1998; Landi *et al.*, 1999; see also Chapter 8).

Independent living

One of the principal claims in the care of older people and individuals with high support needs is that by health and social care organisations working in partnership, individuals can be supported to remain in their own homes for longer. Increased independent living is potentially a very positive outcome for service users and also contributes to efficiency savings, as institutional care tends to cost more than community-based care. The On Lok, Vittorio Veneto and Rovereto evaluations all found that integrated working reduced the cumulative numbers of days older people spent in institutional care. However, in the UK a non-randomised comparative study of an integrated health and social care team found a slight tendency for older people to move in to residential care compared to the control group (Brown *et al.*, 2003). Additionally, this study detected high rates of depression amongst the older people involved, much more so than was predicted at the outset. Jones (2004) suggests that this higher usage of residential care is as a result of agencies working together more closely and sharing more information, thereby lowering the management of risk thresholds for groups with more severe needs than originally predicted. Although this result might not be seen positively (given that usage of residential care was not reduced as expected), this could actually be a better outcome for the individuals concerned who may not otherwise have received appropriate treatment.

Nor is this an isolated example. In the US, the Social HMO demonstration project (see Robinson and Steiner, 1998 for an overview; see also Chapter 3) was associated with increased hospitalisation (although there has been widespread debate about the design of this evaluation; see Leutz *et al.*, 1995, and Kane *et al.*, 1997, for further details). However as Boose (1993) notes, this trend might be explained by better detection rates and follow-up in some of the sites. Again, this demonstrates the importance of evaluating the process of partnership working, looking at how people work together within partnerships and how this differs from traditional services.

Service user satisfaction

Given the trends noted in the previous sections, it might follow that we would expect service user satisfaction to rise as a result. In Australia, the Victoria government initiated a Primary Care Partnership (PCP) strategy which brings together over 800 services in 31 PCPs across all of Victoria. These PCPs seek to improve the experience and outcomes for people who use primary care services and reduce preventable use of acute services through an increasingly preventative approach. The evaluation of this strategy (Australian Institute for Primary Care, 2005) found that PCP service users were more satisfied, felt that services were more coordinated and had not had to repeat information to multiple service providers. The team note that this pattern is found only in the areas where the service coordination tool templates (which are designed to improve the synchronisation of services) were being used. In other words, service users were only getting this improved experience in the areas where these mechanisms were being adopted. The researchers suggest this is evidence that it is these tools which improve service user experience, rather than necessarily the structure of PCP itself or other possible environmental determinants.

Evaluations of the US PACE (Program of All-Inclusive Care for the Elderly) project suggest that it is able to offer highly personalised care, effective clinical coordination and continuity, decreases in hospital/institutional admissions and cumulative days used, and a positive impact on Medicare costs (Kane *et al.*, 1992; Dooley and Zimmerman, 2003). In an earlier section we warned against presuming that service user groups are homogenous. As such, the potential for impact cannot be presumed to be the same for everyone. Despite the improvements the PACE programme produced, Kodner and Kay Kyriacou (2000) note that this service is not suitable for all. Individuals enrolled in this programme had to give up their personal physician which some were not happy with. Moreover, this care programme is delivered within a day-care setting which was also not appropriate for all.

In the UK a study of the first mental health and social care partnership trust (Peck *et al.*, 2002) found that there had been some positive improvements in the mental health status of service users during and immediately after the period of the partnership being established. The research team question whether this can be demonstrated as a consequence of the partnership specifically, or due to wider

environmental changes. The evaluation also included service user satisfaction rat-
ings, but found that there was no statistically significant change in service users'
satisfaction with services across the study period. However, there were three major
areas noted where real problems seemed to exist for mental health service users
in Somerset: level of communication between staff and service users in the process
which led to buildings being closed; the quality of inpatient services; and service
users' knowledge of their care plans. These were not new problems which arose
as a result of the partnership, but had been fairly endemic in the area for a while.
This might lead us to question why it was that a partnership – which took significant staff and managerial time and attention to establish and make work – was
seen as an appropriate way to address these problems. Although Somerset became
renowned within the UK for its innovative services, the experience of some service
users may have been rather different.

Implications and conclusions

Although a variety of different types of impacts have been demonstrated by various
international examples studied in the previous section, none of these are applicable
in a blanket way to all partnerships. Much of the evidence demonstrated above
has come from studies of integrated teams serving distinct populations (usually
older people) which, due to the nature of these services, are more able to construct
randomised or quasi-experimental design methodologies and select clear outcome
indicators relating to functional outcome indicators or cost indicators. Johri *et al.*
(2003) note that effective integrated systems of care of this sort demonstrate three
common features:

- Make use of case management, geriatric assessment and a multidisciplinary
  team.
- Have a single entry point.
- Make use of financial levers (typically through downward substitution of care
  where the team carries the risk this entails, but keeps the financial rewards if
  successful).

However, these lessons are not as widely applicable across all partnerships, and
Johri *et al.* (2003, p. 234) further note that these models have failed to be successfully
generalised on a larger scale. Moreover, the partnership literature is not wholly
positive and suggests some more potentially negative implications. In the Somerset
example (Peck *et al.*, 2002), some buildings were closed down as the new partnership
sought to consolidate its sites. Although this reduced costs and passed on efficiency
savings which could be used to make changes in other areas of the partnership,
those service users who regularly used those buildings might have viewed this as
a negative outcome.

Many of the debates which surround partnership working tend to pertain to
structures and organisational processes. Yet, these types of debates do not often

concern service users directly (who often simply want access to appropriate, timely, high-quality and safe services – regardless of how they are structured). In their study of an integrated health and social care team of older people, Brown *et al.* (2003, p. 93) note:

> It was clearly portrayed ... that users had little interest in who organised or delivered their services as long as they received what they felt they were entitled to. What was of utmost importance was the quality of the relationships which they experienced with service providers at every level of service delivery.

The older people involved in this study were less concerned with how the services were structured, and more concerned that they received the right services to which they were entitled. Clearly this does not apply to all groups of people and there will always be national and regional debates over the appropriate mix of what kinds of organisations provide what care and which mix of staff members should deliver certain types of care. Yet the point remains that if the ultimate goal of partnership is about improving service user outcomes, then we need to be more clear about what kind of outcomes and that these outcomes are the ones which service users want. As Nocon and Qureshi (1996, p. 74) argue, 'it is not enough that measures should be said to be "acceptable" ... Rather, outcome measures must be based on [service users'] own view of the important issues: other approaches are likely to be inappropriate'. A number of studies of integrated teams suggest that they are a more cost-effective way of delivering services (although some commentators have suggested that there is no clear evidence to suggest that team collaboration is more effective than other working methods in terms of cost, e.g. Jenkins, 1999). If partnerships are to be used as a mechanism to lower costs, this is not necessarily a bad thing – they just need to be clear about this intention to all key stakeholders. By being clear about what the partnership is aiming to achieve in terms of partner organisations, staff members and service users, the most appropriate methods may be used to evaluate specific partnerships, using the most appropriate outcome indicators.

Furthermore, the process of surfacing all the outcomes that the partnership is aiming to achieve also holds implications for the nature of partnership working. Once it has been established what the partnership is aiming to achieve, it is important to ensure that a partnership is the best way of achieving this, and if it is, what kind of partnership. As many of the chapters in this text have demonstrated, partnership working is not easy at the best of times, particularly when working within difficult contexts such as those within which health and social care organisations tend to operate. If we are not clear about what we expect from partnerships, we should not be surprised when they fail to deliver. Tools like Theories of Change are useful in assisting the articulation of what partnerships are trying to achieve and also aid the evaluation process.

Partnership working is an international phenomenon which only seems to be expanding in its breadth and scope at the moment. It is central to the modernisation programmes of a number of public sectors around the world, and there is much rhetoric around these mechanisms as ways of improving services for users.

However, if we continue to set unrealistic expectations for these entities, partnerships will inevitably be seen not to have delivered and the concept will lose legitimacy. There is such an extensive partnership literature precisely because, under some circumstances, partnership does seem to be an important mechanism for delivering better services and for tackling complex issues. However, partnership working takes much effort and input from staff members to make effective and if the concept loses legitimacy there is a danger that people will begin to disengage from this process. The outcomes of partnership working are imperative, and it is for this reason that we need to be clear about what kind of working relationships can produce what kind of impacts, for whom, when and why.

Summary

- Outcome measurement is becoming increasingly important in public sector organisations worldwide.
- Despite the prominence of partnerships as potential improvement mechanisms, health and social care partnerships have so far failed to empirically demonstrate that they improve service user outcomes.
- Partnership evaluations have tended to be more concerned with process evaluation than with evaluating the outcomes of partnership working.
- Partnerships are incredibly complex mechanisms to evaluate, and a lack of evidence linking partnerships and improved service user outcomes may be a reflection of this complexity.
- Partnerships internationally have been demonstrated to have impacts on functional and clinical outcome indicators, supporting individuals to live independently and on service user satisfaction.
- The impact that partnerships have is not the same for all partnerships or across service user groups.
- A failure to demonstrate the impact that partnerships have on service users may cause the concept to lose legitimacy in the eyes of staff members and service users.
- It is important that partnerships are clear about what they are trying to achieve.
- Furthermore, it is important that organisations are clear that a partnership is the best possible mechanism to achieve their aims and objectives.

Further reading and useful websites

Helpful sources include:
Dickinson, H. (2008) *Evaluating Outcomes in Health and Social Care*. Bristol, Policy Press.
Dowling, B., Powell, M., and Glendinning, C. (2004) Conceptualising successful partnerships, *Health and Social Care in the Community*, 12, 309–317.
Glendinning, C. et al. (2006) *Outcomes-Focused Services for Older People*. London, SCIE.
Smith, P. (ed.) (1996) *Measuring Outcome in the Public Sector*. London, Taylor & Francis.

Relevant websites include:

The New Zealand government's managing for outcomes programme (http://www.ssc. govt.nz/managing-for-outcomes) includes a tool specifically designed to help organisations consider their progress in results-based management and identify development objectives.

The Canadian government's managing for results self-assessment tool is available via http://www.tbs-sct.gc.ca/rma/account/transmod/tm_e.asp

The UK Department of Health-Funded Social Policy Research Unit at the University of York has a helpful health outcomes programme, with key research reports and tools available via http://www.york.ac.uk/inst/spru/research/summs/outcomes2001–5.htm

The National Council for Voluntary Organisations has some useful resources which define outcomes and suggest how they might be measured: http://www.ncvo-vol.org. uk/

For further information on Theories of Change, see the Aspen Institute Roundtable website: http://www.theoryofchange.org/

For guidance on good practice and on 'what works' in UK health and social care, see the National Institute for Health and Clinical Excellence: http://www.nice.org.uk and the Social Care Institute for Excellence: http://www.scie.org.uk

For general information on partnership evaluation and an example of a partnership evaluation tool, see the POET website: http://hsmcfs3.bham.ac.uk/questionnaire/

References

Australian Institute for Primary Care (2005) *An Evaluation of the Primary Care Partnership Strategy*. Bundoora, Australian Institute for Primary Care.

Barnes, M. *et al.* (2005) *Health Action Zones: Partnerships for Health Equity*. London, Routledge.

Beresford P. *et al.* (2000) Quality in personal social services: the developing role of user involvement in the UK, in C. Davies, L. Finlay and A. Bullman (eds) *Changing Practice in Health and Social Care*. London, Sage.

Bernabei, R. *et al.* (1998) Randomised trial of impact of model of integrated care and case management of older people living in the community, *British Medical Journal*, 316, 1348–1351.

Birckmayer, J.D. and Weiss, C.H. (2000) Theory-based evaluation in practice: what do we learn? *Evaluation Review*, 24, 407–431.

Boose, L. (1993) *A Study of the Differences between Social HMO and Other Medicare Beneficiaries Enrolled in Kaiser Permanente under Capitation Contracts Regarding Intermediate Care Facility User Rates and Expenditures*. Portland, OR, Portland State University.

Brown, L., Tucker, C. and Domokos, T. (2003) Evaluating the impact of integrated health and social care teams on older people living in the community, *Health and Social Care in the Community*, 11, 85–94.

Connell, J.P. *et al.* (Eds.) (1995) *New Approaches to Evaluating Community Initiatives: Concepts, Methods and Contexts*. Washington, DC, The Aspen Institute.

Connell, J.P. and Kubisch, A.C. (1998) Applying a theory of change approach to the evaluation of comprehensive community initiatives: progress, prospects and problems, in K. Fulbright-Anderson, A.C. Kubisch and J.P. Connell (eds) *New Approaches to Evaluating Community Initiatives: Volume 2 – Theory, Measurement and Analysis*. Washington, DC, The Aspen Institute.

Davey, B. *et al.* (2005) Integrating health and social care: implications for joint working and community care outcomes for older people, *Journal of Interprofessional Care*, 19, 22–34.

Department of Health (2006) *Our Health, Our Care Our Say: A New Direction for Community Services*. London, The Stationery Office.

Dickinson, H. (2006) The evaluation of health and social care partnerships: an analysis of approaches and synthesis for the future, *Health and Social Care in the Community*, 14, 375–383.

Dooley, K.J. and Zimmerman, B.J. (2003) Merger as marriage: communication issues in post-merger integration, *Health Care Management Review*, 28, 55–67.

Dowling, B., Powell, M. and Glendinning, C. (2004) Conceptualising successful partnerships, *Health and Social Care in the Community*, 12, 309–317.

Eng, C. *et al.* (1997) Program of all-inclusive care for the elderly (PACE): an innovative model of integrated geriatric care and financing, *Journal of the American Geriatrics Society*, 45, 223–232.

Fulbright-Anderson, K., Kubisch, A.C. and Connell, J.P. (Eds) (1998) *New Approaches to Evaluating Community Initiatives: Theory, Measurement and Analysis*. Washington, DC, Aspen Institute.

Glendinning, C. (2002) Partnerships between health and social services: developing a framework for evaluation, *Policy and Politics*, 30, 115–127.

Hébert, R., Tourigny, A. and Gagnon, M. (2005) *Integrated Service Delivery to Ensure Persons' Functional Autonomy*. Montreal, EDISEM.

HM Treasury (2003) *Every Child Matters*. London, The Stationery Office.

Hood, C. (1991) A public management for all seasons, *Public Administration*, 69, 3–19.

Hudson, B. and Hardy, B. (2002) What is a 'successful' partnership and how can it be measured? in C. Glendinning, M. Powell and K. Rummery (eds) *Partnerships, New Labour and the Governance of Welfare*. Bristol, Policy Press.

Hultberg, E.-L., Lonnroth, K. and Allebeck, P. (2002) Evaluation of the effect of co-financing on collaboration between health care, social services and social insurance in Sweden, *International Journal of Integrated Care*, 2. Available online via http://www.ijic.org

Hultberg, E.-L., Lonnroth, K. and Allebeck, P. (2005) Interdisciplinary collaboration between primary care, social insurance and social services in the rehabilitation of people with musculoskeletal disorder: effects on self-rated health and physical performance, *Journal of Interprofessional Care*, 19, 115–124.

Jenkins, G. (1999) Collaborative care in the United Kingdom, *Primary Care*, 26, 411–422.

Johri, M., Béland, F. and Bergman, H. (2003) International experiments in integrated care for the elderly: a synthesis of the evidence, *International Journal of Geriatric Psychiatry*, 18, 222–235.

Jones, R. (2004) Bringing health and social care together for older people: Wiltshire's journey from independence to interdependence to integration, *Journal of Integrated Care*, 12, 27–32.

Kane, R.L. *et al.* (1997) S/HMOs, the second generation: building on the experience of the first social health maintenance organisation demonstrations, *Journal of the American Geriatrics Society*, 45, 101–107.

Kane, R., Illston, L. and Miller, N. (1992) Qualitative analysis of the program of all-inclusive care for the elderly (PACE), *The Gerontologist*, 32, 771–780.

Kharicha, K. *et al.* (2004) Social work, general practice and evidence-based policy in the collaborative care of older people: current problems and future possibilities, *Health and Social Care in the Community*, 12, 134–141.

Kodner, D.L. and Kay Kyriacou, C. (2000) Fully integrated care for the frail elderly: two American models, *International Journal of Integrated Care*. Available online via http://www.ijic.org

Landi, F. *et al.* (1999) Impact of integrated home care services on hospital use, *Journal of American Geriatric Society*, 47, 1430–1434.

Leutz, W. *et al.* (1995) Medical services in social HMOs: a reply to Harrington *et al.* (letters to the editor), *The Gerontologist*, 35, 6–8.

Nicholas, E., Qureshi, H. and Bamford, C. (2003) *Outcomes into Practice: Focusing Practice and Information on the Outcomes People Value*. York, York Publishing Services.

Nocon, A. and Qureshi, H. (1996) *Outcomes of Community Care for Users and Carers: A Social Services Perspective*. Buckingham, Open University Press.

Office of the Auditor General of Canada (2003) *The Managing for Results Self-Assessment Tool*. Ottawa, Treasury Board of Canada Secretariat.

Ouwens, M. *et al.* (2005) Integrated care programmes for chronically ill patients: a review of systematic reviews, *International Journal for Quality in Health Care*, 17, 141–146.

Peck, E., Gulliver, P. and Towell, D. (2002) *Modernising Partnerships: An Evaluation of Somerset's Innovations in the Commissioning and Organisation of Mental Health Services*. London, Institute of Applied Health and Social Policy, King's College.

Qureshi, H. *et al.* (1998) *Outcomes in Community Care Practice: Number Five*. York, Social Policy Research Unit.

Robinson, R. and Steiner, A. (1998) *Managed Health Care: US Evidence and Lessons for the National Health Service*. Buckingham, Open University Press.

Robson, C. (1993) *Real World Research: A Resource for Real World Scientists and Practitioner-Researchers*. Oxford, Blackwell Publishers Ltd.

Schmitt, M.H. (2001) Collaboration improves the quality of care: methodological challenges and evidence from US health care research, *Journal of Interprofessional Care*, 15, 47–66.

Smith, P. (1996) A framework for analysing the measurement of outcome, in P. Smith (ed.) *Measuring Outcome in the Public Sector*. London, Taylor & Francis.

Thomas, P. and Palfrey, C. (1996) Evaluation: stakeholder-focused criteria, *Social Policy and Administration*, 30, 125–142.

Tourigny, A. *et al.* (2004) Quasi-experimental study of the effectiveness of an integrated service delivery network for the frail elderly, *Canadian Journal on Aging*, 23, 231–246.

Townsley, R., Abbott, D. and Watson, D. (2004) *Making a Difference? Exploring the Impact of Multi-agency Working on Disabled Children with Complex Health Care Needs, Their Families and the Professionals Who Support Them*. Bristol, Policy Press.

Treasury and State Services Commission (2007) *Performance Information Measures and Standards in the SOI and Annual Report*. Wellington, State Services Commission.

Weiss, C.H. (1995) Nothing as practical as good theory: exploring theory-based evaluation for comprehensive community initiatives for children and families, in J.P. Connell *et al.* (eds) *New Approaches to Evaluating Community Initiatives: Concepts, Methods and Contexts*. Washington, DC, The Aspen Institute.

Yordi, C.L. and Waldman, J. (1985) A consolidated model of long-term care: service utilization and cost impacts, *The Gerontologist*, 25, 389–397.

Young, A.F. and Chesson, R.A. (2006) Stakeholders' views on measuring outcomes for people with learning difficulties, *Health and Social Care in the Community*, 14, 17–25.